Advances in Veterinary Oncology

Editor

ANNETTE N. SMITH

VETERINARY CLINICS
OF NORTH AMERICA:
SMALL ANIMAL PRACTICE

www.vetsmall.theclinics.com

September 2014 • Volume 44 • Number 5

ELSEVIER

1600 John F. Kennedy Boulevard • Suite 1800 • Philadelphia, Pennsylvania, 19103-2899
http://www.vetsmall.theclinics.com

**VETERINARY CLINICS OF NORTH AMERICA: SMALL ANIMAL PRACTICE Volume 44, Number 5
September 2014 ISSN 0195-5616, ISBN-13: 978-0-323-32351-2**

Editor: Patrick Manley
Developmental Editor: Susan Showalter

Veterinary Clinics of North America: Small Animal Practice (ISSN 0195-5616) is published bimonthly by Elsevier Inc., 360 Park Avenue South, New York, NY 10010-1710. Months of issue are January, March, May, July, September, and November. Business and Editorial Offices: 1600 John F. Kennedy Blvd., Ste. 1800, Philadelphia, PA 19103-2899. Customer Service Office: 3251 Riverport Lane, Maryland Heights, MO 63043. Periodicals postage paid at New York, NY and additional mailing offices. Subscription prices are $310.00 per year (domestic individuals), $500.00 per year (domestic institutions), $150.00 per year (domestic students/residents), $410.00 per year (Canadian individuals), $621.00 per year (Canadian institutions), $455.00 per year (international individuals), $621.00 per year (international institutions), and $220.00 per year (international and Canadian students/residents). To receive student/resident rate, orders must be accompanied by name of affiliated institution, date of term, and the *signature* of program/residency coordinator on institution letterhead. Orders will be billed at individual rate until proof of status is received. Foreign air speed delivery is included in all *Clinics* subscription prices. All prices are subject to change without notice. **POSTMASTER:** Send address changes to *Veterinary Clinics of North America: Small Animal Practice*, Elsevier Health Sciences Division, Subscription Customer Service, 3251 Riverport Lane, Maryland Heights, MO 63043. Customer Service (orders, claims, online, change of address): Elsevier Periodicals Customer Service, Elsevier Health Sciences Division Subscription Customer Service 3251 Riverport Lane Maryland Heights, MO 63043. Tel: 1-800-654-2452 (U.S. and Canada); 314-447-8871 (outside U.S. and Canada). Fax: 314-447-8029. E-mail: journalscustomerservice-usa@elsevier.com (for print support); journalsonlinesupport-usa@elsevier.com (for online support).

Reprints. For copies of 100 or more of articles in this publication, please contact the Commercial Reprints Department, Elsevier Inc., 360 Park Avenue South, New York, NY 10010-1710. Tel.: 212-633-3874; Fax: 212-633-3820; E-mail: reprints@elsevier.com.

Veterinary Clinics of North America: Small Animal Practice is also published in Japanese by Inter Zoo Publishing Co., Ltd., Aoyama Crystal-Bldg 5F, 3-5-12 Kitaaoyama, Minato-ku, Tokyo 107-0061, Japan.

Veterinary Clinics of North America: Small Animal Practice is covered in *Current Contents/Agriculture, Biology and Environmental Sciences, Science Citation Index, ASCA, MEDLINE/PubMed (Index Medicus), Excerpta Medica,* and *BIOSIS.*

Contributors

EDITOR

ANNETTE N. SMITH, DVM, MS
Diplomate, American College of Veterinary Internal Medicine (Oncology and Small Animal Internal Medicine); Robert and Charlotte Lowder Professor in Oncology, Department of Clinical Sciences, Bailey Small Animal Teaching Hospital, College of Veterinary Medicine, Auburn University, Auburn, Alabama

AUTHORS

JOSEPH W. BARTGES, DVM, PhD
Diplomate, American College of Veterinary Internal Medicine (Small Animal Internal Medicine); DACVN; Department of Small Animal Clinical Sciences, College of Veterinary Medicine, University of Tennessee, Knoxville, Tennessee

PHILIP J. BERGMAN, DVM, MS, PhD
Diplomate, American College of Veterinary Internal Medicine-Oncology; Director, Clinical Studies, VCA, Bedford Hills, New York; Adjunct Associate, Department of Molecular Pharmacology and Chemistry, Memorial Sloan-Kettering Cancer Center, New York, New York

BARBARA BILLER, DVM, PhD
Diplomate, American College of Veterinary Internal Medicine (Oncology); Associate Professor of Oncology, Department of Clinical Sciences, Colorado State University Flint Animal Cancer Center, Fort Collins, Colorado

SARAH BOSTON, DVM, DVSc
Diplomate, American College of Veterinary Surgeons; ACVS Founding Fellow and Associate Professor of Surgical Oncology, Department of Small Animal Clinical Sciences, College of Veterinary Medicine, University of Florida, Gainesville, Florida

BONNIE BOUDREAUX, DVM, MS
Diplomate, American College of Veterinary Internal Medicine (Oncology); Assistant Professor of Medical Oncology, Veterinary Clinical Sciences, Louisiana State University, New Roads, Louisiana

JENNA BURTON, DVM, MS
Diplomate, American College of Veterinary Internal Medicine (Oncology); Assistant Professor of Clinical Oncology, Department of Surgical and Radiologic Sciences, School of Veterinary Medicine, University of California, Davis, Davis, California

JAMES T. CUSTIS, DVM, MS
Diplomate, American College of Veterinary Radiology (Radiation Oncology); Assistant Professor of Radiation Oncology, Department of Environmental and Radiological Health Sciences, Colorado State University Flint Animal Cancer Center, Fort Collins, Colorado

TIMOTHY M. FAN, DVM, PhD
Diplomate, American College of Veterinary Internal Medicine (Oncology, Internal Medicine); Associate Professor, Department of Veterinary Clinical Medicine, University of Illinois at Urbana-Champaign, Urbana, Illinois

RALPH A. HENDERSON Jr, DVM, MS
Diplomate, American College of Veterinary Surgeons; Diplomate, American College of Veterinary Internal Medicine, Oncology; Founding Fellow of Surgical Oncology; Professor Emeritus, Veterinary Surgical Consulting, Auburn, Alabama

CHAND KHANNA, DVM, PhD
Diplomate, American College of Veterinary Internal Medicine (Oncology); Director, Comparative Oncology Program; Head, Tumor and Metastasis Biology Section; Pediatric Oncology Branch, Center for Cancer Research, National Cancer Institute, Bethesda, Maryland

SHAWNA KLAHN, DVM
Assistant Professor, Department of Small Animal Sciences, Virginia-Maryland Regional College of Veterinary Medicine, Virginia Tech, Blacksburg, Virginia

SUSAN M. LARUE, DVM, PhD
Diplomate, American College of Veterinary Surgeons; American College of Veterinary Radiology (Radiation Oncology); Professor of Radiation Oncology, Department of Environmental and Radiological Health Sciences, Colorado State University Flint Animal Cancer Center, Fort Collins, Colorado

CHERYL A. LONDON, DVM, PhD
Diplomate, American College of Veterinary Medicine (Oncology); Director, Clinical Trials Office; Professor, Veterinary Biosciences, The Ohio State University, Columbus, Ohio

DONNA M. RADITIC, DVM, CVA
Diplomate, American College of Veterinary Nutrition; Department of Small Animal Clinical Sciences, College of Veterinary Medicine, University of Tennessee, Knoxville, Tennessee

STEPHANIE E. SCHLEIS, DVM
Diplomate, American College of Veterinary Internal Medicine (Oncology); Clinical Associate Professor of Medical Oncology; Department of Clinical Sciences, Bailey Small Animal Teaching Hospital, Auburn University, Auburn, Alabama

ANNETTE N. SMITH, DVM, MS
Diplomate, American College of Veterinary Internal Medicine (Oncology and Small Animal Internal Medicine); Robert and Charlotte Lowder Professor in Oncology, Department of Clinical Sciences, Bailey Small Animal Teaching Hospital, College of Veterinary Medicine, Auburn University, Auburn, Alabama

Contents

Cancer chemotherapy in dogs and cats has traditionally involved adminis-tration of chemotherapy agents at the maximum tolerated dose. Cytotoxic chemotherapy has an acceptably low risk of serious toxicity, but an oblig-atory rest period must be included to allow for recovery of drug-sensitive normal cell populations. This rest period can also allow significant recovery of tumor cells. Metronomic chemotherapy is characterized by more frequent administration of lower doses of oral drugs and appears to halt or slow tumor progression through multiple mechanisms. This approach may be at least as effective as conventional chemotherapy with a lower risk of toxicity.

Integrative medicine is the combined use of complementary and alter-native medicine with conventional or traditional Western medicine sys-tems. The demand for integrative veterinary medicine is growing, but evidence-based research on its efficacy is limited. In veterinary clinical oncology, such research could be translated to human medicine, be-cause veterinary patients with spontaneous tumors are valuable transla-tional models for human cancers. An overview of specific herbs, botanics, dietary supplements, and acupuncture evaluated in dogs, in vitro canine cells, and other relevant species both in vivo and in vitro is presented for their potential use as integrative therapies in veterinary clinical oncology.

Surgery is a critical component in the treatment of most solid tumors in small animals. Surgery is increasingly combined with adjuvant therapies such as chemotherapy and radiation so surgeons who are treating cancer must have a good understanding of surgical oncology principles, cancer biology, and the roles and potential interactions of surgery, radiation, and chemotherapy. The sequencing plan for these modalities should be determined before treatment is initiated. The surgical oncologist must have a working knowledge of chemotherapy agents and radiation and the effect of these treatments on the ability of tissues to heal and the outcome for the patient.

Cancer is increasingly more common. Several tests for the diagnosis and treatment of cancer in companion animals have been developed. Screening tests discussed include those for lymphoid neoplasia, hemangiosarcoma, and transitional cell carcinoma of the bladder. None of these tests should be used in isolation for diagnosis. Vincristine and doxorubicin are mainstays in the treatment of canine lymphoma. However, it is important and accepted practice to test individuals of predisposed breeds for this mutation before administering these drugs in a lymphoma protocol.

This article discusses the clinically relevant uses of antimicrobials in small animal cancer patients. The article focuses on general considerations of antimicrobial use, antimicrobials in the neutropenic patient, prophylactic antimicrobial usage, antimicrobials in radiation therapy, and antimicrobials in metronomic chemotherapy protocols.

Recent advances in molecular biology have permitted the identification and characterization of specific abnormalities regarding cell signaling and function in cancer cells. Proteins that are found to be dysregulated in cancer cells can serve as relevant targets for therapeutic intervention. Although there are several approaches to block proteins that contribute to cellular dysfunction, the one most commonly used involves a class of therapeutics called small molecule inhibitors. Such inhibitors work by disrupting critical pathways/processes in cancer cells, thereby preventing their ability to grow and survive.

Newer technology, such as intensity-modulated radiation therapy, can dramatically decrease acute radiation side effects, making patients more comfortable during and after treatment. Stereotactic radiation therapy for definitive treatment can be delivered in 1 to 5 fractions, with minimal radiation-associated effects. Image-guided radiation therapy can be used to direct treatment in locations previously not amenable to radiation therapy. Traditional fractionated radiation therapy remains the most commonly available type in veterinary medicine and is the standard of care for many tumors. This article discusses the role of advancements in the treatment of veterinary cancer patients and reviews more traditional radiation treatment.

VETERINARY CLINICS OF NORTH AMERICA: SMALL ANIMAL PRACTICE

THE CLINICS ARE NOW AVAILABLE ONLINE!
Access your subscription at:
www.theclinics.com

Preface

Advances in Veterinary Oncology

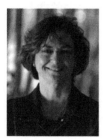

Annette N. Smith, DVM, MS, DACVIM
Editor

This issue of *Veterinary Clinics of North America: Small Animal Practice* examines several topics related to current oncology practice in human and animal patients as well as innovations that have or will become standard of care. Historically, molecular biology was restricted to the research laboratory and had limited contemporaneous application. Currently, targeted therapies, metronomic chemotherapy, therapeutic vaccines, molecular diagnostics, and others are used every day, based on a greater understanding of the mechanisms of cancer development and progression. As information continues to exponentially expand and become more accessible, a basic knowledge of cancer biology and treatment options becomes imperative for every veterinary practitioner. The concept of "one medicine" is maturing into day-to-day reality, and an awareness of clinical trials, as written by Drs Burton and Khanna, is required to best advise our clients about cutting-edge research and options available for their animal companions. Rather than focusing on individual tumor types, these articles present need-to-know broad concepts related to cancer.

Surgery, radiation, and chemotherapy remain mainstays in cancer therapy, but their role is evolving. While surgical excision of tumors is often the first choice of practitioners for diagnosis and treatment, multimodality approaches are frequently important in providing long-term control. Drs Boston and Henderson's article presents the surgical oncologist's view of this reality. Drs LaRue and Custis examine advances in radiation oncology that will provide better tumor control with shorter treatment protocols and decreased side effects. A different use of chemotherapy drugs, so-called "metronomic chemotherapy," is discussed in the article by Dr Biller. Dr London explores the use of the class of chemotherapy agents called small molecule inhibitors, which includes our first veterinary FDA-approved anticancer drug. In addition, Dr Bergman's article on immune strategies includes our first USDA-approved therapeutic cancer vaccine.

Vet Clin Small Anim 44 (2014) xi–xii
http://dx.doi.org/10.1016/j.cvsm.2014.06.004
vetsmall.theclinics.com

Other topics not directly related to cancer treatment, but important in management of our patients, are also presented. Dr Schleis assesses the pros and cons of molecular-based diagnostics for cancer screening and monitoring. The article on neutering and cancer development examines the controversy prompted by several recent articles suggesting a hormonal influence on the occurrence of certain neoplasms. Dr Boudreaux discusses the issue of antibiotic use in the cancer patient, a timely topic given international discussions on the development of problematic drug resistance in both human and veterinary medicine. Dr Fan's article presents strategies for pain management in animals with cancer. Finally, Drs Raditic and Bartges provide evidence for the use of integrative medicine, a growing trend in both human and veterinary patients with cancer.

The last topic, although certainly not least, is Dr Klahn's thorough review of chemotherapy safety for those handling these potentially toxic agents. She has compiled the latest resources for those interested in offering chemotherapy while still maintaining maximal protection for staff and clients that might be exposed. As new laws are enacted and enforced, compliance with these standards will become more important in our practice.

The goal of these articles is to provide familiarity with current oncology concepts to veterinary students and practitioners, although consultation with a veterinary oncologist for the latest information is always advisable, given the rapid evolution of therapeutic strategies. This issue hopefully will establish a solid foundation of knowledge that can be built on as our understanding of cancer continues to expand and new treatments become available. My heartfelt thanks to all of the authors and editors for their invaluable contributions to meeting this objective.

Annette N. Smith, DVM, MS, DACVIM
(Oncology & Small Animal Internal Medicine)
Department of Clinical Sciences
Bailey Small Animal Teaching Hospital
College of Veterinary Medicine
Auburn University
1220 Wire Road
Auburn, AL 36849-5540, USA

E-mail address:
smith30@auburn.edu

Errata

Errors were made in the September 2012 issue (Volume 42, number 5) of *Veterinary Clinics of North America: Small Animal Practice* regarding the exclusion of Dr. Kaoru Endo's name. On page 936 of the article "Interlocking Nails and Minimally Invasive Osteosynthesis", the last sentence leading into page 937 should read as follows:

"Following the successful experimental and clinical use of modified Huckstep nails in animals by Johnson and Huckstep[13] and then Muir and colleagues,[14–16] several dedicated veterinary systems were independently designed in the early 1990s by Dueland and Johnson[17] (United States), Duhautois and van Tilburg[18] (France), Durall and Diaz[19] (Spain), and Endo and colleagues[20] (Japan)."

Likewise, in the same article on page 945, the second sentence of the section "Common Indications" should read:

"During the past 20 years, because of the work of such pioneer surgeons as Johnson,[13] Dueland,[17] Duhautois,[18] Durall,[50] Basinger,[51] Endo,[20] and others, interlocking nailing has gained increasing acceptance in veterinary orthopedics as a reliable osteosynthesis method."

http://dx.doi.org/10.1016/j.cvsm.2014.07.002

In the November 2013 issue (Volume 43, number 6), in the article "Practical Interpretation and Application of Exocrine Pancreatic Testing in Small Animals" by Caroline Mansfield, the statement on page 1250: "This study assessed dogs presenting to an emergency center with signs of acute abdominal disease and found a sensitivity of 82% but a specificity of 59% for SNAP-cPL. Another way of interpreting this is that approximately 40% of dogs with a positive SNAP-cPL had disease other than pancreatitis as their primary presenting problem"

Would more correctly read as:

"This study assessed dogs presenting to an emergency center with signs of acute abdominal disease and found a sensitivity of 82% but a specificity of 59% for SNAP-cPL. Another way of interpreting this is that approximately 40% of dogs without pancreatitis as their primary disease will test positive with the SNAP-cPL."

The author thanks Steve Valeika, DVM, PhD for this correction.

http://dx.doi.org/10.1016/j.cvsm.2014.07.001

---

vetsmall.theclinics.com

Metronomic Chemotherapy in Veterinary Patients with Cancer

Rethinking the Targets and Strategies of Chemotherapy

Barbara Biller, DVM, PhD

KEYWORDS

- Low-dose chemotherapy • Canine neoplasia • Angiogenesis • Immune modulation
- Tumor biomarkers

KEY POINTS

- Metronomic chemotherapy uses old drugs in a new way: at much lower doses and without interruption compared with conventional chemotherapy protocols.
- Rather than targeting the rapidly dividing tumor cell population, metronomic chemotherapy slows or stops tumor growth by inhibiting tumor angiogenesis and evasion from the immune system.
- Most metronomic protocols use oral chemotherapy agents combined with a nonsteroidal antiinflammatory.
- Clinical trials to assess the efficacy of metronomic chemotherapy should include appropriate tumor biomarkers of activity in addition to monitoring changes in tumor volume.

INTRODUCTION

Conventional cytotoxic chemotherapy has been the mainstay of systemic anticancer therapy for more than 50 years. For both human and veterinary patients, most protocols involve administration of single or multiple antiproliferative agents delivered at doses close to the maximum tolerated dose (MTD). Because neoplastic cells are rapidly dividing compared with normal tissues, MTD chemotherapy is intended to kill as much of the neoplastic cell population as possible. A critical aspect of all MTD protocols is inclusion of breaks between drug administrations to allow for

Funding Sources: Morris Animal Foundation (D08CA-054), Zoetis.
Conflict of Interest: None.
Flint Animal Cancer Center, Department of Clinical Sciences, Colorado State University, 300 West Drake Road, Fort Collins, CO 80523-1620, USA
E-mail address: bbiller@colostate.edu

Vet Clin Small Anim 44 (2014) 817–829
http://dx.doi.org/10.1016/j.cvsm.2014.05.003   vetsmall.theclinics.com
0195-5616/14/$ – see front matter © 2014 Elsevier Inc. All rights reserved.

recovery of drug-sensitive normal tissues, particularly bone marrow progenitors and gastrointestinal epithelial cells. Without these gaps between treatments, unacceptable drug toxicities occur. However, this approach also permits recovery of tumor cells and can lead to tumor regrowth and the development of drug-resistant or metastatic disease. Although conventional chemotherapy has been associated with significant gains in survival for many cancers, it infrequently results in permanent tumor control, particularly in the face of demonstrable metastatic disease.

Research over the past several decades has brought about an exponential increase in understanding of the molecular pathways and mechanisms of cancer metastasis and drug resistance. This work has revealed many reasons for the failure of conventional chemotherapy to limit cancer progression. These reasons include the dynamic heterogeneity and instability of tumor cells, the protective action of the tumor microenvironment, and suppression of antitumor immune responses. However, awareness of these shortcomings is enabling the development of more targeted approaches to cancer therapy including a form of chemotherapy known as metronomic chemotherapy (MC). In contrast with conventional chemotherapy, MC is characterized by the continuous or uninterrupted administration of chemotherapy drugs at doses that are significantly lower than MTD therapy (**Box 1**).[1] As discussed in this article, MC can be thought of as a multitargeted approach and is rapidly emerging as an attractive adjunct or alternative to conventional drug delivery. Although many questions regarding the application of MC to human and veterinary oncology patients await investigation, favorable tumor control and excellent safety profiles support the significant promise of this new anticancer approach.

TARGETS OF MC
Tumor Angiogenesis

Tumor growth is critically dependent on the process of angiogenesis, which occurs through the development of new blood vessels from preexisting, larger vessels. Tumors can also stimulate vasculogenesis, which is defined as new blood vessel formation from bone marrow–derived progenitor cells including circulating endothelial progenitor cells (CEPs).[2–4] Regardless of the pathway, the rapidly dividing tumor cell population requires a blood supply to deliver nutrients and oxygen and to remove waste products; without it, tumor volume is limited to only a few millimeters in size.[5,6]

Box 1
Key differences between conventional chemotherapy and MC

- Conventional chemotherapy uses large doses of drugs that target the rapidly dividing tumor cell population

- Because conventional chemotherapy also kills rapidly dividing cells of the bone marrow and gastrointestinal tract, a break between treatments is necessary to prevent serious toxicity

- MC uses much lower doses of chemotherapy drugs given without any breaks between treatments; the dose is generally too low to kill tumor cells directly

- The targets of MC include the tumor vasculature and certain immune cells that help tumor cells hide from recognition and attack by the immune system

- The success of conventional chemotherapy is based on a significant decrease in tumor volume; treatment responses to MC are often based on achievement of durable stable disease

Because angiogenesis is so important to their survival, tumors are adept at disrupting the normal balance between proangiogenic and antiangiogenic molecules that characterizes the physiologic angiogenesis of organ system development, wound healing, and other normal processes. Also referred to as the angiogenic switch, tumor formation drives the upregulation of a large number of growth factors, including vascular endothelial growth factor (VEGF), fibroblast growth factor, and platelet-derived growth factor (PDGF). Of these, VEGF is most important, stimulating angiogenesis through direct effects on endothelial cell proliferation and migration and through mobilization of CEPs from the bone marrow to sites of neovascularization.[7,8]

The other important aspect of the angiogenic switch is tumor-induced inhibition of naturally occurring antiangiogenic molecules such as thrombospondin-1 (TSP-1). Inhibition of TSP-1 activity is an effective tumor survival strategy because TSP-1 has direct suppressive effects on endothelial cell proliferation and apoptosis and is therefore a potent VEGF antagonist.[9] In human patients with cancer, increased serum or intratumor concentrations of VEGF and decreased levels of TSP-1 are associated with poor outcome for many malignancies, including carcinomas of lung, breast, and bladder.[10,11]

Although it may seem surprising, drugs from nearly every class of conventional chemotherapy agents have been found to have antiangiogenic activity based on the results of various in vitro and in vivo assays.[12,13] Similar to the neoplastic cell population, the endothelial cells recruited to support tumor growth are also rapidly dividing and as such are susceptible to cytotoxic chemotherapy.[13] Some drugs, including vinblastine and paclitaxel, inhibit endothelial cell proliferation at doses lower than those required to inhibit tumor cell proliferation.[14,15] Why then are the antiangiogenic effects of MTD chemotherapy not more clinically relevant? The answer to this question arises from the discovery by Browder and colleagues[16] that the long, but necessary, break periods between MTD dosing permit regrowth and recovery of damaged tumor vasculature at a pace that outweighs any benefit of the drugs' antiangiogenic effects. When the alkylating agent cyclophosphamide (CYC) (Cytoxan) was given at the MTD to mice with lung cancer, apoptosis of endothelial cells in the tumor vasculature occurred even before tumor cell death did. However, this antiangiogenic activity had no therapeutic benefit because damage to the vasculature was repaired during the recovery periods between successive cycles of chemotherapy. When CYC was given at a lower dose (about one-third of the MTD in these studies) and without interruption, then even large, well-established tumors were found to regress.[16]

Since this ground-breaking work many preclinical studies have confirmed the antiangiogenic effects of metronomic dosing of CYC and other chemotherapy agents. Some drugs, such as the microtubule inhibitors vinblastine and paclitaxel, inhibit endothelial cell proliferation or migration directly.[15,17,18] Other drugs, including CYC and 5-fluorouracil, seem to have additional indirect antiangiogenic effects through mechanisms including decreased mobilization of CEPs and induction of TSP-1 and other endogenous angiogenic inhibitors.[19–22] The combined effects of metronomic drug delivery with other antiangiogenic agents such as cyclooxygenase (COX)-2 and receptor tyrosine kinase inhibitors is an area of active investigation. The rationale for their evaluation is based on the finding that blockade of COX-2 and tyrosine kinase receptors overexpressed on many neoplastic cells disrupts the aberrant intracellular signaling cascade that leads to production of VEGF, PDGF, and other proangiogenic growth factors.[23,24] Combination of MC with other agents such as bevacizumab (Avastin), a monoclonal antibody that binds to VEGF, and trastuzumab (Herceptin), an antibody that targets human ErbB-2 receptors, is also being explored.[25,26] These agents are designed to be administered on a frequent and long-term basis, making their combination with MC a logical choice. Although preliminary, accumulating evidence supports the notion that the combination of antiangiogenic agents with different mechanisms of action may be synergistic.[27]

The antiangiogenic effects of MC on canine tumors are largely unknown. In a clinical trial of dogs with soft tissue sarcoma, oral administration of CYC at 15 mg/m^2/d was associated with a significant decrease in tumor microvessel density within 14 days based on serial tumor biopsies.[28] At lower doses (10 and 12.5 mg/m^2/d) there was no change in blood vessel density in the tumor biopsies. This study did not evaluate other potential biomarkers of angiogenesis such as VEGF levels and circulating endothelial cells (CECs). In a more recent study the administration of low-dose CYC to mice with canine malignant melanoma xenografts had no impact on tumor microvessel density unless combined with the nonsteroidal antiinflammatory drug (NSAID) piroxicam (Feldene).[29] This drug combination also decreased intratumor secretion of VEGF while increasing expression of TSP-1. Although preliminary, these studies suggest that metronomic delivery of CYC interferes with canine tumor angiogenesis and support the concept that combination of MC with an NSAID may increase efficacy.

Tumor Immunology

The ability of tumors to grow undetected by the body's immune system is a key feature of the tumorigenic process. An environment that favors immune suppression rather than activation helps neoplastic cells evade attack by cytotoxic and helper T cells and natural killer cells. A central tactic is tumor-induced recruitment of immunosuppressive regulatory T lymphocytes (T$_{reg}$) and myeloid derived suppressor cells (MDSCs). T$_{reg}$ and MDSCs have important roles in limiting pathologic inflammation under physiologic conditions. In patients with cancer, T$_{reg}$ and MDSCs efficiently suppress antitumor immune responses, thereby helping to establish tumor tolerance and facilitate the development of metastatic disease.[30-32] Other immune cells, such as dendritic cells and macrophages, also contribute to immune suppression through changes in their activation phenotype and secretion of antiinflammatory rather than proinflammatory cytokines.[32]

Recent investigation has uncovered a growing number of conventional chemotherapy drugs that display both immunostimulatory and immune-suppressive effects, a difference that sometimes depends only on the dose and schedule of drug administration. High-dose CYC, for example, has long been used as a myeloablative and lymphoablative preconditioning therapy for procedures such as bone marrow transplant and adoptive T-cell transfer.[33,34] A single intravenous dose of CYC at 500 to 650 mg/m^2 (about 2-fold higher than the dose used for conventional chemotherapy) is given before bone marrow transplant in dogs with lymphoma. This dose induces a transient but profound neutropenia, lymphopenia, and thrombocytopenia within 7 days of administration.[35]

In contrast, metronomic dosing of CYC is associated with multiple immunostimulatory effects, including decreases in the number and function of T$_{reg}$, dendritic cell activation, and stimulation of cytotoxic T cells.[36] In mouse tumor models and in humans with advanced cancer, low-dose CYC has been shown to increase the efficacy of immunotherapy and at least partially restore antitumor immune responses.[37,38] The alkylating agents CYC and chlorambucil may also have immunostimulatory effects in tumor-bearing dogs. In 2 separate investigations of dogs with soft tissue sarcoma, administration of either CYC at 15 mg/m^2/d or chlorambucil at 0.1 mg/kg/d led to a decrease in the number of T$_{reg}$ in peripheral blood compared with baseline control values.[28,39] In another study, metronomic CYC in combination with the tyrosine kinase inhibitor toceranib (Palladia) led to an increase in serum concentrations of the proinflammatory cytokine interferon gamma, suggesting improvement in cytotoxic T cell function.[40] Low, noncytotoxic concentrations of other agents including pacli-taxel, doxorubicin, methotrexate, and gemcitabine have also been shown to improve antitumor immunity through various mechanisms such as dendritic cell activation, improvement of cytotoxic T-cell function, and reduction of MDSC activity.[41–43] As un-derstanding of the immunomodulatory effects of chemotherapy agents continues to grow, combination of MC with tumor immunotherapy is expected to become an area of active investigation for veterinary patients.

Other Potential Targets

Tumor dormancy is an evolutionary stage of tumor development in which residual cancer cells are present but inactive as a result of cell cycle arrest or equilibrium be-tween apoptosis and proliferation.[44] In tandem with this phenomenon is the recent discovery of cancer stem cells or tumor initiating cells, a tumor cell phenotype with characteristic self-renewal capabilities distinct from the main tumor cell population. Some experimental data suggest that cancer stem cells and dormant tumor cells reside in close proximity to the tumor vasculature, thus increasing their susceptibility to antiangiogenic agents.[45] For example, in mice with glioma or hepatocellular carcinoma, antiangiogenic therapy led to apoptosis of cancer stem cells and induc-tion of tumor dormancy.[46,47] Whether this potential mechanism of action will trans-late into a therapeutic benefit for human or veterinary patients awaits further investigation.

CLINICAL TRIALS INVESTIGATING MC
Summary of Human Clinical Trials

About 10 years ago the results of a landmark clinical trial were reported in which 64 women with metastatic breast cancer received daily low-dose CYC and twice-weekly methotrexate. This study found a disease control rate (complete remission, partial remission, or durable stable disease) of 32% and a low incidence (13%) of mod-erate leukopenia.[48] Because most of the women had already been treated with and had failed MTD chemotherapy protocols containing CYC, these results sparked signif-icant interest in further investigation of MC for the treatment of advanced cancers.

Since this time favorable results have been reported for a wide range of malig-nancies encompassing solid tumors and hematologic neoplasms. A recent systematic review of fully published clinical trials in humans yielded 80 studies involving mainly heavily pretreated patients with advanced or metastatic carcinomas of breast, pros-tate, lung, intestines, and liver.[49] All were either phase I or II studies and most involved small numbers of patients (60 or fewer). Overall, the mean disease control rate was an impressive 56% and the incidence of serious toxicity was very low (8%). A few studies for other malignancies such as melanoma, sarcoma, glioblastoma and lymphoma have also been described.[50] Most trials to date have evaluated administration of metronomic CYC, either alone or in combination with other chemotherapy agents or antiangiogenic therapies such as the NSAID celecoxib (Celebrex) or the anti-VEGF monoclonal antibody bevacizumab.[49] There are also several ongoing phase III trials in which the efficacy of MC is being explored either as a maintenance therapy following adjuvant MTD chemotherapy or as an alternative to MTD protocols in human breast or colorectal carcinoma.[51] **Table 1** provides a summary of key findings from some of the larger and most recent clinical trials.

Despite the promising disease control rates and a low incidence of toxicity, MC is still considered investigational and generally is not offered as first-line therapy. A survey of

Table 1
Results of typical human clinical trials evaluating MC

Tumor Type	Drugs Used	Number of Patients	Study Design	Overall Clinical Benefit (%)[a]
Metastatic breast cancer[69]	Oral CYC + methotrexate	90	Prospective/ randomized	41.5
Metastatic breast cancer	Oral CYC + methotrexate + trastuzumab[b]	22	Prospective	46
Refractory ovarian cancer[70]	Oral CYC + bevacizumab	70	Prospective	24
Refractory prostate cancer[71]	Oral CYC + celecoxib	29	Retrospective	45
Pediatric sarcomas[72]	Oral CYC + vinorelbine	18	Prospective	41
Relapsed lymphoma[73]	Oral CYC + celecoxib	35	Prospective	37
Relapsed multiple myeloma[74]	Oral CYC + prednisone + thalidomide	37	Prospective	63

[a] The overall clinical benefit was defined as the percentage of patients with an objective response or durable stable disease (usually longer than 6 months).
[b] Trastuzumab is a monoclonal antibody that targets the HER2/neu receptor, which is overexpressed on many human breast cancers.
    Data from Refs.[69–74]

medical oncologists in Europe found that MC is typically prescribed after failure of at least 2 previous lines of treatment.[52] However, dosing and frequency of metronomic protocols is often determined empirically, making evaluation of efficacy and comparisons between protocols difficult. As more trial results are reported, a better of understanding of proper patient selection, drug combinations, and monitoring strategies seems likely to advance MC toward the front line of therapy for some malignancies.

Veterinary Clinical Trials

MC is an attractive treatment option in veterinary patients for many reasons, including ease of drug administration, reasonable cost, and lower toxicity profile compared with MTD chemotherapy protocols. Thus far there have been 9 published reports of clinical trials investigating metronomic drug delivery in dogs and cats with cancer, and these are summarized in **Table 2**. All have been either phase I or phase II and most have prospectively evaluated MC in the face of gross disease. As in human trials, MC seems well tolerated and there is early evidence of favorable tumor responses. Although major questions concerning efficacy, patient selection, chronic toxicity, drug dosing, combinations, and so forth await further investigation, MC is rapidly becoming a popular treatment option.

MC IN CLINICAL PRACTICE: CHALLENGES AND FUTURE DIRECTIONS
Biomarkers for MC

One of the biggest hurdles in the application of MC to clinical practice is the lack of readily available biomarkers to monitor response to therapy; predict patients most likely to respond; and to aid in determination of the proper dose, frequency, and duration of treatment. In contrast with MTD chemotherapy, in which a measurable change

Table 2
Published clinical trials evaluating MC in dogs and cats

Tumor Type	Chemotherapy Drug	Dose	Other Drugs	n/Species	Outcome	Comments
Hemangiosarcoma[53]	CYC	12.5–25 mg/m^2 daily for 3 wk (alternating with etoposide)	Etoposide 50 mg/m^2 daily for 3 wk, piroxicam daily 0.3 mg/kg	9/Dogs	Median DFI (178 d); comparable with DFI for MTD doxorubicin	Toxicity less than for MTD chemotherapy but 15% developed SHC
Soft tissue sarcoma[54]	CYC	10 mg/m^2 daily or every other day	Piroxicam daily 0.3 mg/kg	30/Dogs	Median DFI (>410 d) greater than surgery alone (211 d)	12% of dogs developed SHC
Soft tissue sarcoma[28]	CYC	12.5 mg/m^2 daily or 15 mg/m^2 daily	None	11/Dogs	N/A	Evaluated T_{reg}# and tumor angiogenesis
Multiple types[59]	CYC	25 mg/m^2 daily	Celecoxib daily 2 mg/kg	15/Dogs	40% OCB[a]	Evaluated MC as first line vs metastatic disease
Multiple types[40]	CYC	15 mg/m^2 daily	Toceranib 2.75 mg/kg every other day	15/Dogs	N/A	Evaluated T_{reg}# and other immune effects
Multiple types[58]	CYC	Approximately 14 mg/m^2 daily or every other day	Most on COX inhibitors	24/Cats	88% OCB	No serious toxicities
Multiple types[57]	Lomustine	2.84 mg/m^2 daily	None	81/Dogs	36% OCB	27% had to stop treatment because of toxicity
Multiple types[55]	Chlorambucil	4 mg/m^2 daily	None	36/Dogs	58% OCB	No serious toxicities
TCC of bladder[56]	Chlorambucil	4 mg/m^2 daily	Most on COX inhibitors	31/Dogs	67% OCB	No serious toxicities

Abbreviations: DFI, disease-free interval; n, number enrolled; N/A, not assessed; OCB, overall clinical benefit; SHC, sterile hemorrhagic cystitis; TCC, transitional cell carcinoma; T_{reg}#, Number of regulatory T cells (T_{reg}).

[a] The OCB was defined as the percentage of patients with an objective response or stable disease with variable duration.

Data from Refs.[28,40,53–59]

in tumor volume is the most important criteria in determination of response, the goal of MC is often to achieve durable stable disease. Therefore successful clinical trial design depends critically on identification of appropriate biomarkers and study end points.

Most of the research in veterinary oncology has been focused on identification of biomarkers of angiogenesis. In a recent study by Marchetti and colleagues,[59] determination of baseline plasma VEGF levels by enzyme-linked immunosorbent assay (ELISA) was predictive of response to MC in dogs with metastatic neoplasia. This finding is consistent with similar studies in humans in which pretreatment VEGF and TSP-1 levels predict response to antiangiogenic therapy and prognosis for patients with cancer of the breast and lungs.[10,60] However, simple comparison of pretreatment and posttreatment VEGF or TSP-1 levels may be unreliable because detection of antiangiogenic activity does not necessarily correspond with decreases in tumor volume.

Detection of CECs and CEPs in the blood of patients with cancer may serve as one of the most useful surrogate markers of angiogenesis and of antiangiogenic drug therapy.[3,61] In mice and humans, CECs and CEPs have also been used to identify the optimal biological activity of metronomic drug dosing.[62,63] However, debate continues as to the phenotype of these rare cell populations, and their accurate detection depends on access to a flow cytometer and other sophisticated equipment.[64]

Canine CECs and CEPs have been identified and isolated from whole blood.[65] This method was applied to the monitoring of treatment responses in dogs with soft tissue sarcoma given 1 of 2 synthetic mimetic peptides of TSP-1 (known as ABT-510 and ABT-898).[66] Although CECs could be measured in serial blood samples obtained during treatment, there was no change in total mean CEC values, and baseline CECs levels were not useful in delineation of the responding and nonresponding patient populations. For MC protocols using CYC, dose optimization may be more feasible by measuring changes in numbers of circulating T_{reg} over time. This finding was suggested by the work of Burton and colleagues,[28] which showed a dose-dependent reduction in T_{reg} numbers during metronomic CYC administration in dogs with soft tissue sarcoma.

Side Effects

The results of clinical studies in humans show that MC is well tolerated, causing only mild to moderate toxicity in most studies.[49,50] Thus far, this seems to be the case in dogs. Despite these observations it is important to remember that MC has risks and that some drugs or drug combinations may have unanticipated toxicities in addition to their effects on angiogenesis or the antitumor immune response. For example, combination of MC with antiangiogenic agents such as bevacizumab or receptor tyrosine kinase inhibitors may increase the risk of hypertension, edema, proteinuria, and diarrhea in human patients.[51]

Experience with combination therapy is limited in veterinary oncology but is a new area of investigation. In a recent study of dogs receiving toceranib, the addition of metronomic CYC did not seem to increase the incidence of toxicity.[40] In this prospective clinical trial CYC was not introduced until any side effects of toceranib administration were well controlled. Although the incidence of adverse events was low during the 8-week study period, the potential toxicity of more chronic drug administration was not evaluated. However, the risk for the development of sterile hemorrhagic cystitis may be greater with cumulative CYC administration and seems equally likely with either metronomic or MTD chemotherapy.[67] As with any chemotherapy treatment plan, appropriate monitoring for potential toxicity should continue to be a routine part of patient care.

Development of Drug Resistance

At first, the potential for the development of resistance to MC was thought to be low based on the genetic stability of endothelial cells compared with the mutation-prone tumor cell targeted by MTD chemotherapy.[12] However, evidence for the development of resistance to MC therapy is accumulating. Recent work in a mouse model of hepatocellular carcinoma revealed that a residual population of tumor cells remained in the liver following metronomic CYC therapy.[47] Despite disappearance of gross disease and a significant decrease in the number of tumor cells in circulation, the residual tumor cells expressed characteristics of tumor stem cells and were ultimately responsible for the development of hepatic metastases. Of particular concern are reports of the increased invasive and metastatic abilities of MC-resistant tumor stem cells compared with the primary tumor cell population.[68] This process, known as metastatic conditioning, has been observed as a consequence of antiangiogenic therapy in several preclinical models. Further investigation into the factors related to metastatic conditioning as well as drug resistance patterns of MC are ongoing.

Practical Guidelines for Veterinary Patients with Cancer

Although MC is an attractive treatment choice, it is still considered an experimental approach with the potential for toxicity. When available, conventional therapies should first be offered before turning to a metronomic protocol. Because stable disease is generally the goal of therapy it is also important to consider the overall condition of the patient; living with stable disease should be expected to result in an acceptable quality of life. When used appropriately there is much potential for MC to improve, not just maintain, quality of life for companion animals with cancer, especially as additional studies answer important questions regarding indications, drug dosages, and patient monitoring.

SUMMARY

MC represents an important shift in thinking about the targets and the strategies of cancer chemotherapy. By targeting key tumor-associated survival pathways such as angiogenesis and immune escape, MC may be both more effective and less toxic than conventional chemotherapy. As understanding of tumor biology, immunology, and other components of the tumor microenvironment continues to grow, MC protocols and clinical trials will become better justified, designed, and monitored. These results will provide a new opportunity to combine MC with other anticancer therapies and to improve the outcome for humans and animals with cancer.

REFERENCES

1. Hanahan D, Weinberg RA. The hallmarks of cancer. Cell 2000;100:57–70.
2. Asahara T, Murohara T, Sullivan A, et al. Isolation of putative progenitor endothelial cells for angiogenesis. Science 1997;275:964–7.
3. Bertolini F, Shaked Y, Mancuso P, et al. The multifaceted circulating endothelial cell in cancer: towards marker and target identification. Nat Rev Cancer 2006;6: 835–45.
4. Bertolini F, Mancuso P, Kerbel RS. Circulating endothelial progenitor cells. N Engl J Med 2005;353:2613–6 [author reply: 2613–6].
5. Folkman J. Angiogenesis in cancer, vascular, rheumatoid and other disease. Nat Med 1995;1:27–31.

6. Folkman J. Tumor angiogenesis: therapeutic implications. N Engl J Med 1971; 285:1182–6.
7. Rafii S, Lyden D, Benezra R, et al. Vascular and haematopoietic stem cells: novel targets for anti-angiogenesis therapy? Nat Rev Cancer 2002;2:826–35.
8. Brantley-Sieders DM, Fang WB, Hicks DJ, et al. Impaired tumor microenvironment in EphA2-deficient mice inhibits tumor angiogenesis and metastatic progression. FASEB J 2005;19:1884–6.
9. Lawler PR, Lawler J. Molecular basis for the regulation of angiogenesis by thrombospondin-1 and -2. Cold Spring Harb Perspect Med 2012;2:a006627.
10. Fleitas T, Martinez-Sales V, Vila V, et al. VEGF and TSP1 levels correlate with prognosis in advanced non-small cell lung cancer. Clin Transl Oncol 2013;15: 897–902.
11. Shariat SF, Youssef RF, Gupta A, et al. Association of angiogenesis related markers with bladder cancer outcomes and other molecular markers. J Urol 2010;183:1744–50.
12. Kerbel RS, Kamen BA. The anti-angiogenic basis of metronomic chemotherapy. Nat Rev Cancer 2004;4:423–36.
13. Miller KD, Sweeney CJ, Sledge GW Jr. Redefining the target: chemotherapeutics as antiangiogenics. J Clin Oncol 2001;19:1195–206.
14. Vacca A, Iurlaro M, Ribatti D, et al. Antiangiogenesis is produced by nontoxic doses of vinblastine. Blood 1999;94:4143–55.
15. Belotti D, Vergani V, Drudis T, et al. The microtubule-affecting drug paclitaxel has antiangiogenic activity. Clin Cancer Res 1996;2:1843–9.
16. Browder T, Butterfield CE, Kraling BM, et al. Antiangiogenic scheduling of chemotherapy improves efficacy against experimental drug-resistant cancer. Cancer Res 2000;60:1878–86.
17. Wang J, Lou P, Lesniewski R, et al. Paclitaxel at ultra low concentrations inhibits angiogenesis without affecting cellular microtubule assembly. Anticancer Drugs 2003;14:13–9.
18. Pasquier E, Tuset MP, Street J, et al. Concentration- and schedule-dependent effects of chemotherapy on the angiogenic potential and drug sensitivity of vascular endothelial cells. Angiogenesis 2013;16:373–86.
19. Vizio B, Novarino A, Giacobino A, et al. Pilot study to relate clinical outcome in pancreatic carcinoma and angiogenic plasma factors/circulating mature/progenitor endothelial cells: preliminary results. Cancer Sci 2010;101: 2448–54.
20. Damber JE, Vallbo C, Albertsson P, et al. The anti-tumour effect of low-dose continuous chemotherapy may partly be mediated by thrombospondin. Cancer Chemother Pharmacol 2006;58:354–60.
21. Bocci G, Francia G, Man S, et al. Thrombospondin 1, a mediator of the antiangiogenic effects of low-dose metronomic chemotherapy. Proc Natl Acad Sci U S A 2003;100:12917–22.
22. Ooyama A, Oka T, Zhao HY, et al. Anti-angiogenic effect of 5-fluorouracil-based drugs against human colon cancer xenografts. Cancer Lett 2008; 267:26–36.
23. Gately S, Kerbel R. Therapeutic potential of selective cyclooxygenase-2 inhibitors in the management of tumor angiogenesis. Prog Exp Tumor Res 2003;37: 179–92.
24. Shibuya M. Vascular endothelial growth factor and its receptor system: physiological functions in angiogenesis and pathological roles in various diseases. J Biochem 2013;153:13–9.

25. Mayer EL, Isakoff SJ, Klement G, et al. Combination antiangiogenic therapy in advanced breast cancer: a phase 1 trial of vandetanib, a VEGFR inhibitor, and metronomic chemotherapy, with correlative platelet proteomics. Breast Cancer Res Treat 2012;136:169–78.
26. Francia G, Man S, Lee CJ, et al. Comparative impact of trastuzumab and cyclophosphamide on HER-2-positive human breast cancer xenografts. Clin Cancer Res 2009;15:6358–66.
27. Kerbel RS. Reappraising antiangiogenic therapy for breast cancer. Breast 2011; 20(Suppl 3):S56–60.
28. Burton JH, Mitchell L, Thamm DH, et al. Low-dose cyclophosphamide selectively decreases regulatory T cells and inhibits angiogenesis in dogs with soft tissue sarcoma. J Vet Intern Med 2011;25:920–6.
29. Choisunirachon N, Jaroensong T, Yoshida K, et al. Effects of low-dose cyclophosphamide with piroxicam on tumour neovascularization in a canine oral malignant melanoma-xenografted mouse model. Vet Comp Oncol 2013. [Epub ahead of print].
30. Toh B, Abastado JP. Myeloid cells: prime drivers of tumor progression. Oncoimmunology 2012;1:1360–7.
31. Umansky V, Sevko A. Tumor microenvironment and myeloid-derived suppressor cells. Cancer Microenviron 2013;6(2):169–77.
32. Finn OJ. Immuno-oncology: understanding the function and dysfunction of the immune system in cancer. Ann Oncol 2012;23(Suppl 8):viii6–9.
33. Dudley ME, Wunderlich JR, Yang JC, et al. Adoptive cell transfer therapy following non-myeloablative but lymphodepleting chemotherapy for the treatment of patients with refractory metastatic melanoma. J Clin Oncol 2005;23:2346–57.
34. Dudley ME, Yang JC, Sherry R, et al. Adoptive cell therapy for patients with metastatic melanoma: evaluation of intensive myeloablative chemoradiation preparative regimens. J Clin Oncol 2008;26:5233–9.
35. Lane AE, Chan MJ, Wyatt KM. Use of recombinant human granulocyte colony-stimulating factor prior to autologous bone marrow transplantation in dogs with lymphoma. Am J Vet Res 2012;73:894–9.
36. Penel N, Adenis A, Bocci G. Cyclophosphamide-based metronomic chemotherapy: after 10 years of experience, where do we stand and where are we going? Crit Rev Oncol Hematol 2012;82:40–50.
37. Ge Y, Domschke C, Stoiber N, et al. Metronomic cyclophosphamide treatment in metastasized breast cancer patients: immunological effects and clinical outcome. Cancer Immunol Immunother 2012;61:353–62.
38. Ghiringhelli F, Menard C, Puig PE, et al. Metronomic cyclophosphamide regimen selectively depletes CD4+CD25+ regulatory T cells and restores T and NK effector functions in end stage cancer patients. Cancer Immunol Immunother 2007;56:641–8.
39. Back A, Schleis S, Smith A, et al. The evaluation of CD4+CD25+FoxP3+ regulatory T-cells before and one month after metronomic chlorambucil in dogs with soft tissue sarcoma. Veterinary Cancer Society 2013 Annual Conference. Minneapolis, MN, October 18, 2013. p. 137.
40. Mitchell L, Thamm DH, Biller BJ. Clinical and immunomodulatory effects of toceranib combined with low-dose cyclophosphamide in dogs with cancer. J Vet Intern Med 2012;26:355–62.
41. Nars MS, Kaneno R. Immunomodulatory effects of low dose chemotherapy and perspectives of its combination with immunotherapy. Int J Cancer 2013;132: 2471–8.

42. Shurin GV, Tourkova IL, Kaneno R, et al. Chemotherapeutic agents in noncyto-
    toxic concentrations increase antigen presentation by dendritic cells via an IL-
    12-dependent mechanism. J Immunol 2009;183:137–44.
43. Suzuki E, Kapoor V, Jassar AS, et al. Gemcitabine selectively eliminates splenic
    Gr-1+/CD11b+ myeloid suppressor cells in tumor-bearing animals and en-
    hances antitumor immune activity. Clin Cancer Res 2005;11:6713–21.
44. Aguirre-Ghiso JA. Models, mechanisms and clinical evidence for cancer
    dormancy. Nat Rev Cancer 2007;7:834–46.
45. Calabrese C, Poppleton H, Kocak M, et al. A perivascular niche for brain tumor
    stem cells. Cancer Cell 2007;11:69–82.
46. Folkins C, Man S, Xu P, et al. Anticancer therapies combining antiangiogenic
    and tumor cell cytotoxic effects reduce the tumor stem-like cell fraction in glioma
    xenograft tumors. Cancer Res 2007;67:3560–4.
47. Martin-Padura I, Marighetti P, Agliano A, et al. Residual dormant cancer stem-
    cell foci are responsible for tumor relapse after antiangiogenic metronomic ther-
    apy in hepatocellular carcinoma xenografts. Lab Invest 2012;92:952–66.
48. Colleoni M, Rocca A, Sandri MT, et al. Low-dose oral methotrexate and cyclo-
    phosphamide in metastatic breast cancer: antitumor activity and correlation
    with vascular endothelial growth factor levels. Ann Oncol 2002;13:73–80.
49. Lien K, Georgsdottir S, Sivanathan L, et al. Low-dose metronomic chemo-
    therapy: a systematic literature analysis. Eur J Cancer 2013;49:3387–95.
50. Romiti A, Cox MC, Sarcina I, et al. Metronomic chemotherapy for cancer treat-
    ment: a decade of clinical studies. Cancer Chemother Pharmacol 2013;72:13–33.
51. Loven D, Hasnis E, Bertolini F, et al. Low-dose metronomic chemotherapy: from
    past experience to new paradigms in the treatment of cancer. Drug Discov
    Today 2013;18:193–201.
52. Collova E, Sebastiani F, De Matteis E, et al. Use of metronomic chemotherapy in
    oncology: results from a national Italian survey. Tumori 2011;97:454–8.
53. Lana S, U'Ren L, Plaza S, et al. Continuous low-dose oral chemotherapy for
    adjuvant therapy of splenic hemangiosarcoma in dogs. J Vet Intern Med
    2007;21:764–9.
54. Elmslie RE, Glawe P, Dow SW. Metronomic therapy with cyclophosphamide and
    piroxicam effectively delays tumor recurrence in dogs with incompletely re-
    sected soft tissue sarcomas. J Vet Intern Med 2008;22:1373–9.
55. Leach TN, Childress MO, Greene SN, et al. Prospective trial of metronomic
    chlorambucil chemotherapy in dogs with naturally occurring cancer. Vet
    Comp Oncol 2012;10:102–12.
56. Schrempp DR, Childress MO, Stewart JC, et al. Metronomic administration of
    chlorambucil for treatment of dogs with urinary bladder transitional cell carci-
    noma. J Am Vet Med Assoc 2013;242:1534–8.
57. Tripp CD, Fidel J, Anderson CL, et al. Tolerability of metronomic administration
    of lomustine in dogs with cancer. J Vet Intern Med 2011;25:278–84.
58. Leo C. Evaluation of low-dose metronomic (LDM) cyclophosphamide toxicity in
    cats with malignant neoplasia. J Feline Med Surg 2014. [Epub ahead of print].
59. Marchetti V, Giorgi M, Fioravanti A, et al. First-line metronomic chemotherapy in
    a metastatic model of spontaneous canine tumours: a pilot study. Invest New
    Drugs 2012;30:1725–30.
60. Ioachim E, Damala K, Tsanou E, et al. Thrombospondin-1 expression in breast
    cancer: prognostic significance and association with p53 alterations, tumour
    angiogenesis and extracellular matrix components. Histol Histopathol 2012;
    27:209–16.

61. Farace F, Massard C, Borghi E, et al. Vascular disrupting therapy-induced mobilization of circulating endothelial progenitor cells. Ann Oncol 2007;18:1421–2.
62. Montagna E, Cancello G, Bagnardi V, et al. Metronomic chemotherapy combined with bevacizumab and erlotinib in patients with metastatic HER2-negative breast cancer: clinical and biological activity. Clin Breast Cancer 2012;12:207–14.
63. Calleri A, Bono A, Bagnardi V, et al. Predictive potential of angiogenic growth factors and circulating endothelial cells in breast cancer patients receiving metronomic chemotherapy plus bevacizumab. Clin Cancer Res 2009;15: 7652–7.
64. Mancuso P, Bertolini F. Circulating endothelial cells as biomarkers in clinical oncology. Microvasc Res 2010;79:224–8.
65. Wills TB, Heaney AM, Jane Wardrop K, et al. Immunomagnetic isolation of canine circulating endothelial and endothelial progenitor cells. Vet Clin Pathol 2009;38:437–42.
66. Sahora AI, Rusk AW, Henkin J, et al. Prospective study of thrombospondin-1 mimetic peptides, ABT-510 and ABT-898, in dogs with soft tissue sarcoma. J Vet Intern Med 2012;26:1169–76.
67. Gaeta R, Brown D, Cohen R, et al. Risk factors for development of sterile haemorrhagic cystitis in canine lymphoma patients receiving oral cyclophosphamide: a case-control study. Vet Comp Oncol 2012. [Epub ahead of print].
68. Paez-Ribes M, Allen E, Hudock J, et al. Antiangiogenic therapy elicits malignant progression of tumors to increased local invasion and distant metastasis. Cancer Cell 2009;15:220–31.
69. Colleoni M, Orlando L, Sanna G, et al. Metronomic low-dose oral cyclophosphamide and methotrexate plus or minus thalidomide in metastatic breast cancer: antitumor activity and biological effects. Ann Oncol 2006;17:232–8.
70. Orlando L, Cardillo A, Ghisini R, et al. Trastuzumab in combination with metronomic cyclophosphamide and methotrexate in patients with HER-2 positive metastatic breast cancer. BMC Cancer 2006;6:225.
71. Fontana A, Bocci G, Galli L, et al. Metronomic cyclophosphamide in elderly patients with advanced, castration-resistant prostate cancer. J Am Geriatr Soc 2010;58:986–8.
72. Casanova M, Ferrari A, Bisogno G, et al. Vinorelbine and low-dose cyclophosphamide in the treatment of pediatric sarcomas: pilot study for the upcoming European Rhabdomyosarcoma Protocol. Cancer 2004;101:1664–71.
73. Buckstein R, Kerbel RS, Shaked Y, et al. High-dose celecoxib and metronomic "low-dose" cyclophosphamide is an effective and safe therapy in patients with relapsed and refractory aggressive histology non-Hodgkin's lymphoma. Clin Cancer Res 2006;12:5190–8.
74. Suvannasankha A, Fausel C, Juliar BE, et al. Final report of toxicity and efficacy of a phase II study of oral cyclophosphamide, thalidomide, and prednisone for patients with relapsed or refractory multiple myeloma: a Hoosier Oncology Group Trial, HEM01-21. Oncologist 2007;12:99–106.

Evidence-based Integrative Medicine in Clinical Veterinary Oncology

Donna M. Raditic, DVM, CVA*, Joseph W. Bartges, DVM, PhD

KEYWORDS

- Complementary and alternative medicine • Integrative medicine
- Veterinary oncology • Cancer • Neoplasia • Dietary supplements • Herbs
- Nutraceutical

KEY POINTS

- There is a growing demand for use of integrative medicine in veterinary clinical oncology.
- Evidence-based research on using integrative medicine in veterinary clinical oncology is scarce.
- Translational research with animal models of human cancers is an opportunity to expand the knowledge of the etiopathogenesis of neoplasia and identify treatments.
- Metabolomics research may provide the evidence-based research needed to accelerate the use of complementary and alternative medicine in both human and veterinary oncology.

Integrative medicine (IM) is the use of complementary and alternative medicine (CAM) with conventional Western medicine systems. CAM therapies include herbs, supplements, acupuncture, massage, and others that are rational and supported by evidence to alleviate physical and emotional symptoms, improve quality of life (QOL), and possibly improve adherence to oncology treatment regimens. Demand for IM is growing, and veterinarians are being challenged to know more about these therapies.[1,2]

Herbs and dietary supplements (HDS) are the most accessible form of CAM. Reportedly, more than half of the human population used HDS between 2003 and 2006. In 2010, US herbal supplement sales exceeded $5.2 billion.[3] Between 20% and 55% of human patients with cancer use HDS. Specifically, 67% to 87% of women with breast cancer and those 9 years after diagnosis use supplements. One study reported that 67% of clients gave their pets with cancer HDS, indicating commonplace use.[4]

The authors have no financial disclosures to acknowledge.
Department of Small Animal Clinical Sciences, College of Veterinary Medicine, University of Tennessee, 2407 River Drive, Knoxville, TN 37996, USA
* Corresponding author.
E-mail address: draditic@utk.edu

Vet Clin Small Anim 44 (2014) 831–853
http://dx.doi.org/10.1016/j.cvsm.2014.06.002   vetsmall.theclinics.com
0195-5616/14/$ – see front matter Published by Elsevier Inc.

In treating a patient with cancer being given supplements, veterinarians face multiple questions and challenges, the most important being safety and efficacy. Veterinarians must rely on scientific evidence but cannot overlook the client's perspective. Reportedly, human oncology patients use natural products to empower themselves, attempt to take control of their health, and increase QOL.[3] Considering the strength of the human-animal bond, logically pet owners would apply these same emotions.[5] Owners use supplements, herbs, massage, and acupuncture in their own health care, so they expect veterinarians to have a basic understanding of CAM, especially with respect to cancer, chronic illnesses, and geriatrics.

Knowledgeable patients value physicians who embrace them as empowered participants in making their own health care decisions. The health care provider in this shifted perspective is an informed intermediary, an expert guide, and a consultant to the patient. The Society of Integrative Oncology in 2009 outlined guidelines for IM as part of cancer care. The Clinical Practice Committee outlined best recommendations for curcumin, glutamine, Vitamin D, maitake mushrooms, fish oils, green tea, milk thistle, Astragalus, melatonin, and probiotics.[3]

If a veterinarian is not responsive and knowledgeable about CAM, owners will likely seek advice from friends, nonprofessional literature, and the Internet, which provide ample but possibly incorrect information. In 2005, 60% of veterinarians reported that they needed skills or knowledge related to CAM on a weekly or monthly basis and 7% indicated situations arose daily. CAM is incorporated less into veterinary curricula than in medical schools.[6]

Evidence-based research on CAM in an IM plan in veterinary clinical oncology is scarce, which is expected because large-scale research funding is typically provided for projects with potential for profits, such as with new, patented drugs. Still, value exists in assessing current literature and exploring IM that either has potential or is already based on evidence for use in veterinary oncology with respect to growth of translational research and the "One Health" movement.

Animal models of human cancers are an opportunity to help both veterinary and human patients by expanding the knowledge of the pathogenesis of neoplasia and identifying specific treatments. Pets live in the same environments as humans and eat similar foods, thus are exposed to similar risk factors; therefore, the etiopathogenesis of canine and feline tumors is likely similar to that of human tumors. For example, breast cancer is the most common malignancy in women, and the mammary gland is a common site for tumor development in bitches.[7]

Veterinary pilot studies can justify investment of sizable resources required to complete larger trials, especially when positive results are documented in an animal model. In preclinical studies of cancer therapeutics, important information could be acquired for new and innovative therapies. Advantages are that dogs develop cancer about twice as frequently as humans, and the presentation, histology, and biology of many canine cancers closely parallel human cancers. In addition, body size of dogs simplifies biologic sampling, whereas shorter overall lifespan allows for spontaneous development and course of disease within a time frame reasonable for data collection.[8]

Cancer is an important disease in dogs and accounts for 27% of all deaths in purebred dogs in the United Kingdom. Without reliable historical tumor registries, it is difficult to know whether prevalence of cancer in dogs is increasing. However, animals are living longer as a result of improvements in health care, and cancer is generally a disease of older age.[7] Also, advances in veterinary medicine, particularly diagnostics, and higher owner expectations are likely to result in increased diagnosis. Focus on QOL comes to the forefront of a veterinary treatment plan because the patient has a shorter lifespan than a human, and economics of treatment is different. With a diagnosis of cancer comes an opportunity to explore an IM approach in veterinary clinical oncology, as illustrated by the pilot trial using *Coriolus versicolor* mushroom extract in treatment of canine hemangiosarcoma.[8]

Quantitatively measuring the dynamic, multiparametric metabolic responses of living systems to pathophysiological stimuli or genetic modification (metabolomics) may be an avenue to develop evidence-based research for the use of IM. Recent metabolomic studies have demonstrated significant potential of IM in areas such as responses to environmental stress, toxicology, nutrition, global effects of genetic manipulation, cancer, diabetes, disease diagnosis, and natural product discovery. A major benefit of metabolomics is that profiling can usually be achieved by noninvasively examining urine or plasma samples with proton nuclear magnetic resonance (NMR) spectroscopy, high-power liquid chromatography, and mass spectroscopy for biomarkers that could detect early-stage disease, identify residual disease postsurgery, and help to monitor response and detect early toxicity.[9] Interestingly, one of the goals of metabolomics studies is identifying discrete patterns and specific treatments in oncology patients, which parallels IM's emphasis on the individual, known as "patient-centered care." Combining translational medicine and metabolomics research may spawn rapid development in veterinary oncology.

Ideally, an integrative approach to veterinary clinical oncology should target many physiologic and biochemical tumor pathways while minimizing normal tissue toxicity and supporting overall QOL. The oncologist should first *primum non nocere*, or do no harm, while weighing risks and benefits of conventional treatment. Integrating CAM must be done *non nocere* with consideration of evidence of available research.

Because of the lack of formal education regarding IM in veterinary medical curricula and sparse research, the authors consulted with experienced veterinarians who use CAM to determine what is being used clinically in integrative veterinary oncology (Erin Bannink, DVM, DACVIM [oncology], Bloomfield Hills, MI, personal communication, 2013; and Steve Marsden, DVM, ND, MSOM, L.Ac, Dipl. CH, RH [AGH], Edmonton, Alberta, Canada, personal communication, 2013).[10] The evidence base for the use of relevant HDS was assessed via a literature search for uses of HDS in the dog/cat, in vitro using dog/cat cells, and then in other species, including humans or in vitro cell lines. No meta-analysis and few randomized controlled clinical trials (RCCT) using supplements in veterinary oncology were found. Reports on use of HDS in feline oncology and feline cells are minimal.

HERBS/BOTANICS EVALUATED IN DOGS OR IN VITRO CANINE CELLS

Few herbs or botanic extracts have been evaluated in RCCTs in dogs and canine cancer cells. The *C versicolor* mushroom, commonly referred to as cloud mushroom, turkey tail, or Yunzhi mushroom in China, contains polysaccharopeptide (PSP), which causes cell-cycle arrest at the G_1/S checkpoint with alterations in apoptogenic and extracellular signaling proteins. The net result is a reduction in proliferation and an increase in apoptosis in cancer cells.[11,12] One randomized, double-blind, multidose pilot study examined I'm-Yunity, a proprietary fractionation of *C versicolor* mushroom extract (Integrated Chinese Medicine Holdings, Ltd., Hong Kong, China), in 15 splenectomized dogs with a histopathologic diagnosis of splenic hemangiosarcoma. Median time to development or progression of abdominal metastases was significantly delayed in dogs receiving 100 mg/kg/d I'm-Yunity (112 days; range 30–308 days) compared with dogs receiving 25 mg/kg/d (30 days; range 16–126 days; $P = .046$), but was not significantly different than in dogs receiving 50 mg/kg/d; however, there was no placebo group. No adverse events were reported.[8]

Another study used a standardized formulation of maitake (*Grifola frondosa*) mushroom extract (Maitake PETfraction; PureFormulas, Medley, FL) in 15 dogs with intermediate-grade and high-grade lymphoma. Although the extract was well-tolerated and induced no negative effects, no decrease greater than 50% (objective response) in lymph node size occurred in 13 of 15 dogs.[13]

Skorupski and colleagues[14] examined the protective effects of a combination of S-adenosylmethionine (SAMe) and silybin (Denamarin; Nutramax Laboratories, Edgewood, MD) for lomustine (CCNU)-induced hepatotoxicity in 50 dogs. SAMe is found naturally in the body, and silybin is a flavonolignan of milk thistle (*Silybum marianum*).[15] In this study, cancer-bearing dogs with normal alanine aminotransferase (ALT) activities were randomized to receive CCNU ($\pm$ corticosteroids) alone or with concurrent Denamarin, and plasma biochemical analysis was performed before each dose. More dogs receiving CCNU alone had an increase in ALT compared with dogs receiving CCNU with Denamarin (84% vs 68%). Denamarin is often recommended for dogs prescribed CCNU, because hepatocellular damage is likely decreased and the chance of completing a course of chemotherapy is increased.[14]

Canine high-grade B-cell lymphoma is often used as a model for human non-Hodgkin lymphoma. Because epidemiologic studies indicate that soy-containing diets are associated with a lower incidence of many human tumors, an in vitro study using 2 canine B-cell lymphoid cell lines evaluated genistein (4,5,7-trihydroxyisoflavone), a readily available isoflavone found in soy-based products, and genistein-combined polysaccharide (GCP). Both genistein and GCP led to cell death via apoptosis, and the treated cells exhibited increased Bax:Bcl-2 ratios.[16] GCP was also found to inhibit cell proliferation, increase apoptosis, and induce G_2/M arrest in 3 human and 4 canine lymphoid cell lines.[17] However, an in vivo, dose-escalating pharmacokinetic study determined that therapeutic serum levels of genistein were not reached with oral dosing of GCP in normal dogs.[16]

In an in vitro study in canine osteosarcoma D-17 cells, treatment with α-mangostin, a xanthone derived from the mangosteen fruit (*Garcinia mangostana*), resulted in nuclear condensation and fragmentation, typical of apoptosis.[18] Other reported antitumor effects are in human breast and prostate cancer and leukemia.[19]

HERBS/BOTANICS EVALUATED IN VIVO OR IN VITRO IN OTHER SPECIES

A few in vivo and in vitro studies in other species demonstrate effects of herbs and their antitumor mechanisms. However, most of these treatments seldom progress to quality multi-institutional RCCTs that evaluate response rate and survival. **Table 1** lists some herbs that have been evaluated for their anticancer effects and seem targeted for more research.

Some studies, including human pharmacokinetic studies, have been performed with extracts of herbs, including curcumin, ginseng, ginkgo, ginger, and milk thistle.[20] Curcumin has been reported to influence many cell signaling pathways involved in tumor initiation and proliferation. Its use has been limited because of low bioavailability, which has been overcome with recent innovations in encapsulation and nanoparticles; the herb can now be found in combination formulas such as ProstaCaid and BreastDefend (ecoNugenics, Santa Rosa, CA).[21,22]

Hydrophobic flavonoids from *Scutellaria baicalensis* and the polyphenol honokiol from *Magnolia officinalis* have undergone in vivo and in vitro studies. The former has been evaluated in skin cancer, pancreatic cancer, lymphoma, myeloma, lung cancer, and carcinoma, with reported antitumor mechanisms such as oxidative radical scavenging, attenuation of NF-$\kappa\beta$ activity, inhibition of gene regulation of the cell cycle, and

Table 1
Herbs that have been evaluated in vivo and/or in vitro in species other than dogs

Herb	Active Ingredients	Modes of Action
Angelica (Korean *Angelica gigas* Nakai)	Decursin, decursinol	Decreased angiogenesis, inhibition of VEGF
Artemisinin (*Artemisia annua,* Chinese wormwood)	Artemisone, artesunate, dihydroartemisinin	Apoptosis, decreased NF-κB, inhibition VEGF, chemosensitization, reduced MMPs
Astragalus (*Astragalus membranaceus*)	Bioactive polysaccharide, flavonoids, calycosin	Cell-mediated immune mechanisms stimulated, MDR reversal, inhibition of VEGF and HIF-1α
Atractylodes	Bioactive polysaccharides, lactone	Inhibition of proteolysis inhibiting factor, reduction of cytokines
Boswellia (frankincense)	Boswellic acid (ABKA and KBA)	Anti-inflammatory, inhibition of MMP and leukotrienes
Bupleurum (*Radix Bupleuri*)	Saikosaponins	Increased Fas/Fas ligand apoptotic system, inhibition of COX-2 and reactive oxygen species (ROS)-mediated apoptosis
Carthamus	Safflower polysaccharide	Apoptosis, increased cytotoxic NK cells
Coptis	Berberine	Bax/Bcl-2 apoptosis, activation of caspase and PARP
Curcumin (*Curcuma longa*)		Inhibition of COX-2, cyclin D1, and MMPs; inhibition of NF-κB, STAT, and TNF-α signaling; p53 expression regulation; inhibition of I3K/akt signaling
Gingko biloba	Flavonoid glycosides	Increased free-radical scavengers systems (SOD, catalase, glutathione)
Ginseng (*Panax ginseng*)	Ginsenosides	Immunomodulation, activated p53, inhibition of NF-κB, ROS generation
Ginger (*Zingiber officinale*)	6-shogaol, acetoxychavicol acetate, terpenes	Decreases chemotherapy-induced nausea and vomiting, apoptosis via p53 and caspase 3, down-regulation of anti-apoptotic proteins, inhibition of NF-κB and TNF-α, increased antioxidant enzymes SOD, catalase, and GPx

(*continued on next page*)

Table 1
(continued)

Herb	Active Ingredients	Modes of Action
Licorice (*Glycyrrhiza glabra*)	Isoliquiritigenin (phenol)	Inhibition of VEGF and MMP 2,9
Magnolia (*M officinalis*)	Magnolol, lignin, honokiol polyphenol	Apoptosis via cleavage of caspase 8 and PARP; inhibition of HIF-1α, VEGF, AMPK, MMP 2,9, and histone deacetylases; decreased COX2, PGEα, and TNF-α
Milk thistle (*S marianum*)	Silybin (flavonoid), silibinin (flavonolignan)	Enhanced expression of TNF-related apoptosis-inducing ligand death receptors; inhibition of NF-κB & VEGF
Mistletoe (*Viscum album*)	Mistletoe lectin	Acts as pattern-recognizing ligands activates T-cell response against cancer cells
Panax notoginseng	Ginsenosides (protopanaxadiol and panaxydol)	Hemostasis, apoptosis, G_1 phase arrest, caspase 3 activation
Rehmannia	Acteoside (phenylpropanoid glycoside)	Down-regulation of tyrosinase activity, activation of p53 apoptosis, decreased TNF-α and IL1-β
Skullcap (*S baicalensis*, Chinese skullcap)	Baicalin, wogonin hydrophilic flavonoids	Apoptosis via PI3K/akt signaling, inhibition of IL-6, decreased MMP-2

Abbreviations: ABKA, 3-O-acetyl-11-keto-beta-boswellic acid; Akt, cytosolic protein kinase; AMPK, adenosine monophosphate-activated protein kinase; Bax/Bcl-2, Bcl-2 associated X protein/B-cell lymphoma-2; COX-2, cyclooxygenase-2; GPx, glutathione peroxidase; HIF-1α, Hypoxia inducible factor 1 alpha; IL1-β, interleukin (IL)-1b beta; IL-6, interleukin-6; KBA, 11-Keto-β-boswellic acid; MDR, multidrug resistance; MMP, matrix metalloproteinase; NF-κB, nuclear factor kappa-light chain enhancer of activated B-cells; PARP, poly-ADP ribose polymerase; PGEα, prostaglandin E2 alpha; SOD, superoxide dismutase; STAT, signal transducer and activator of transcription; TNF-α, tumor necrosis factor alpha; VEGF, vascular endothelial growth factor.
Data from Refs.[15,23,25–27,32,102–162]

suppression of cyclooxygenase-2 (COX-2) gene expression with almost no effects on normal cells.[23–25] Bladder, lung, skin, and breast cancer research (in vivo and in vitro) has evaluated mechanisms of honokiol.[26]

Milk thistle, with the active ingredient silibinin, a flavonolignan, has been studied in colon, prostate, and lung cancers. It is also being developed into topical and injectable formulations,[27] demonstrating that preparations may be standardized, safety margins known, and research and marketing can be successful.

BIOACTIVE POLYSACCHARIDES: FUNGI

β-ᴅ-Glucans, now termed bioactive polysaccharides, are high-molecular-weight, complex branch-chained polysaccharides found especially in fungi with specific configurations of β1-3, 1-4, or 1-6 branch chains, which have been shown to have immunostimulating activities. The importance of their structure-function relationship has been reported in studies looking at their immunomodulating activity, including activation of macrophages, monocytes, natural killer (NK) cells, dendritic cells (DCs), and lymphocytes. These bioactive polysaccharides have been shown to have antitumor effects in lung, breast, cervical, and prostate cancer, and melanoma.[28]

Immunomodulating activity has been shown to be due to glucan receptors on cell surfaces, such as monocytes and other immune cells. Fungal polysaccharides, such as *Agaricus blazei, Cordyceps sinensis, Ganoderma* species, and *G frondosa*, have been systematically studied for development into nutraceuticals and include established drugs polysaccharide-K (PSK, Krestin; Kureha Chemicals Industry Corp., Tokyo, Japan) from *Trametes versicolor* (Tv mushrooms), and lentinan from *Lentinus edodes*. Variable bioactivity may be due to differences in receptor affinity or receptor-ligand interaction. The immunomodulation action is via differing receptors involving dectin-1, toll-like receptors (TLR), and an increase of antioxidant capacity.[28]

A phase I/II dose escalation study using orally administered preparations from Tv in 9 women with breast cancer after standard chemotherapy and radiotherapy concluded that up to 9 g/d was safe and tolerable in the immediate posttreatment setting and may improve immune status in immunocompromised patients with breast cancer.[29] A larger phase I/II dose escalation trial of 32 postmenopausal patients with breast cancer free of disease after initial treatment was performed using a maitake liquid extract. The primary endpoints were safety and tolerability, but the study demonstrated a statistically significant association between maitake and immunologically stimulatory and inhibitory measurable effects in peripheral blood.[30]

A meta-analysis of 5 RCCT studies evaluated clinical and adverse effects of *Ganoderma lucidum* in patients with cancer. The following parameters were described: tumor response, evaluated according to the World Health Organization criteria; immune function parameters, such as NK cell activity; and QOL, measured by the Karnofsky scale. Patients who had been given *G lucidum* with chemo/radiotherapy were more likely to respond, whereas *G lucidum* treatment alone did not demonstrate the same regression rate as that seen in combined therapy, supporting its use as an adjunct to conventional treatment. The results suggested that *G lucidum* potentially stimulates host immunity and tumor response, but concluded uncertainty in enhancement of long-term survival.[31]

These bioactive polysaccharides possess other antitumor properties whose exact mechanisms are unknown, such as stimulation of cell differentiation, hematopoiesis, antimetastasis, and anti-angiogenesis.[32,33] A direct and/or synergistic response in tumor regression has been shown in animal studies with mammary carcinoma, metastatic lung metastasis, gastric carcinoma, and melanoma.[34,35] It is possible that specific glucans have a role in triggering complement-dependent antitumor cytotoxicity. A synergistic effect with tumor regression was evident with administration of β-D-glucans together with monoclonal antibodies against GD2 ganglioside, G250 protein, and CD20 protein in experimental neuroblastoma, carcinoma, and CD20+ lymphoma, respectively.[36]

The turkey tail mushroom (*C versicolor, T versicolor*) is one of the most studied mushrooms, with extracts such as PSK, PSP, Tv polysaccharides, and versicolor polysaccharide affecting different cancer cell lines.[37] Peer-reviewed publications on their antitumor effects include 37 in vitro articles, 55 animal studies, 43 human clinical studies, and 11 review articles in gastrointestinal, breast, and lung cancer. In vitro data suggest that the immunologic effects of PSK are mediated through TLR (transverse cell membrane proteins located on DCs and macrophages) and stimulation of TNF secretion; they are TLR-4-dependent, but dectin-1 independent. These innate immune cells respond to foreign invaders and at the same time trigger the release of inflammatory cytokines that activate T and B cells. TLRs link innate and active immunity in a specific recognized role.

A meta-analysis of PSK trials in colorectal cancer showed a positive impact on clinical outcomes. Tv is standard for oncology treatment in mainstream, modern Japanese cancer management, and PSK was approved in 1977 as a cancer therapy by the Japanese National Health Registry. It now represents 25% of the total national costs of cancer care in Japan.[37]

Three randomized trials (n = 227, 376, 914 women) evaluated PSK immunotherapy (3000 mg/d) in patients with breast cancer. PSK treatment resulted in significantly extended survival times when added to standard protocols, or comparable survivals to conventional chemotherapy.[37] At the time of this writing, the National Institutes of Health/National Center for CAM was considering funding for a breast cancer clinical trial using PSK, with collaboration between Fred Hutchinson/University of Washington Cancer Consortium and Bastyr University.

ACUPUNCTURE

Acupuncture involves the stimulation of A delta nerve fibers, which then activate interneurons in the dorsal horn of the spinal cord; produce encephalins and other endogenous opioids, anti-inflammatory cytokines, and neuropeptides; and may also inhibit C nerve fibers in the dorsal horn. An abundance of animal studies is published suggesting acupuncture for analgesic use, but the clinical evidence from RCCTs in noncancer patients has not been able to demonstrate that acupuncture is conclusively superior to sham acupuncture for analgesia.[2,38] Currently, there are no studies on acupuncture in dogs or cats with cancer, but human studies suggest benefits in pain management, anorexia, gastrointestinal effects, and QOL.

Research in human acupuncture demonstrates potential uses for specific cancer-related complications. In a breast cancer study evaluating upper limb lymphedema, postsurgical arm circumference improved in acupuncture-treated patients.[39,40] Similarly, in another study using acupressure in human patients with colorectal cancer, there was shortened time to first flatus passage and oral liquid intake, and improved gastrointestinal function in patients after abdominal surgery.[41]

Overall, the literature supports the use of acupuncture for cancer-related pain management, but concern is repeatedly expressed about methodology and sampling bias.[42,43] One review suggested protocols generated from RCCTs should be adopted by clinicians using acupuncture and that clinicians should possess knowledge and skills in both acupuncture and allopathic oncology.[38]

Several studies support the use of acupuncture to treat chemotherapy-induced nausea/vomiting, but a need for more research and repeatable protocols is emphasized. These studies evaluated acupressure, electro-acupuncture, as well as traditional acupuncture.[1,44] Defining specific endpoints and study designs are issues with studies evaluating acupuncture for cancer-related fatigue and QOL.[45]

DIETARY SUPPLEMENTS EVALUATED IN DOGS OR IN VITRO CANINE CELLS AND RELEVANT STUDIES IN OTHER SPECIES OR IN VITRO

A 2004 review of nutrition and supplements as complementary therapy in pets with cancer included the following key nutritional factors: soluble carbohydrate, fiber, protein, arginine, fat, and omega-3 (N-3) fatty acids (FAs). It also includes a brief discussion of nutraceuticals, including antioxidant vitamins, trace minerals, glutamines, protease inhibitors, garlic, tea polyphenol, vitamin A, and shark cartilage.[5] More current studies looking at these and other nutrients and their role in cancer in the dog and canine cell lines are evaluated in later discussion.

Calcitriol

Calcitriol (1,25-dihydroxycholecalciferol; 1α25-dihydroxycholecalciferol), the principal biologically active form of vitamin D, exerts potent antineoplastic activity in vitro and in vivo in a broad range of tumor model systems. Calcitriol induces G_1/G_0 cell-cycle arrest and apoptosis, while down-regulating Bcl-2, decreasing epidermal growth factor, and inhibiting tumor invasion through decreased metalloproteinase (MMP)-2 and metalloproteinase-9 activity.[46,47] Calcitriol was synergistic with cisplatin using in vitro canine tumor cells and a phase I clinical study to determine the maximum tolerated dose (MTD) of this combination in dogs with cancer and to characterize the pharmacokinetics of calcitriol in dogs.[47] An open-label, single-dose, 2-way crossover study with dogs randomly receiving calcitriol either intravenously or orally, followed by cisplatin, demonstrated a lower MTD of cisplatin when receiving calcitriol in 10 tumor-bearing dogs studied. Conclusions were that high-dose oral calcitriol has moderate bioavailability and individual variability is similar to that reported in humans. Serum levels in some dogs were at the level shown to have antitumor activity in a preclinical murine model.[48]

Calcitriol exhibits synergistic, antiproliferative in vitro activity when used with other chemotherapeutics, including CCNU, vinblastine, imatininib, or toceranib. A study using canine mastocytoma C2 cells reported calcitriol increases chemotherapy or tyrosine kinase inhibitor cytotoxicity. The study also used a highly concentrated formulation of calcitriol as a single therapy in dogs with mast cell tumors. Remission was obtained in 4 of 10 dogs, but the study was discontinued because of adverse events.[49]

Calcitriol inhibited canine transitional cell carcinoma cells via G_0/G_1 cell-cycle arrest.[50] Calcitriol has also been shown to inhibit proliferation and induce apoptosis in 2 types of human bladder cancer cells and N-methyl nitrosourea–induced rat tumors.[51] Recent studies demonstrate that the antiproliferative effects of calcitriol are mediated by the nuclear vitamin D receptor (VDR), with one study reporting improved survival associated with an increase in VDR expression in lung adenocarcinoma cells.[52]

Retinoids

Retinoids are needed for normal cell signaling, and studies have evaluated this vitamin for cancer protection and treatment. Retinoids are used to treat cancers via their actions on cell differentiation, proliferation, and apoptosis. In humans, retinoids are used in treatment of acute promyelytic leukemia (APL), medulloblastoma, and metastatic melanoma. They enhance effects of chemotherapeutics such as cisplatin in ovarian carcinoma, squamous head and neck cancers, hepatoma, and lung and breast cancers. The primary limitation of the use of retinoids is retinoid resistance, which is well identified in APL.[53]

A 42% response rate to retinoid treatment has been seen in dogs with cutaneous lymphoma, and positive results have been seen with in vitro canine mast cells and osteosarcoma cell lines.[54] Numerous clinical studies are using new and synthetic retinoids, alone or in combination therapy, for the treatment of breast, ovarian, renal, head and neck, melanoma, and prostate cancers in human oncology; overall, results continue to be promising.[53,55,56]

Antioxidants

Use of antioxidants in oncology patients has been controversial. It has been hypothesized that selenium supplementation exerts an anticarcinogenic effect by reducing the naturally occurring genotoxic stress within the aging prostate. In a translational RCCT using 49 intact male elderly beagles, the extent of DNA damage in prostate cells and in peripheral blood lymphocytes was lower among the selenium-supplemented dogs.[57] In another randomized study, data from elderly beagles being supplemented with selenium as a model for prostate cancer were compared with data from 2 humans. Six markers of prostatic homeostasis that likely contribute to prostate cancer risk reduction were measured in the aged beagles—intraprostatic dihydrotestosterone (DHT), testosterone (T), DHT:T, epithelial cell DNA damage, proliferation, and apoptosis.[58]

The human literature suggests a decrease in peripheral neuropathy associated with paclitaxel with vitamin E, glutamine, and L-carnitine supplementation. Vitamin E with glutamine decreased severity of oral mucositis resulting from radiation and chemotherapy, and glutamine and probiotics can reduce chemotherapy-induced diarrhea.[59] Vitamin E delta-tocotrienol significantly enhanced the efficacy of gemcitabine to inhibit pancreatic cancer growth and survival in vitro and in vivo.[60]

A review of antioxidant use in 19 studies using Cochrane Collaboration methodology[61] found no evidence of significant decreases in chemotherapy efficacy. Another review of antioxidants that evaluated glutathione, melatonin, vitamin A, and an antioxidant mixture of N-acetylcysteine, vitamin E, selenium, L-carnitine, and Co-Q10 reported either decreased chemotherapy toxicity or no difference with the supplementation of all antioxidants examined except one study of vitamin A, which resulted in increased toxicity.[62] A systematic review of antioxidant use in gastrointestinal cancers appeared to show an increase in overall mortality.[63] Vitamins A, C, E, and selenium, alone or in different combinations, did not prevent lung cancer nor decrease lung cancer mortality, but some evidence showed a small increase in lung cancer mortality in smokers or persons exposed to asbestos and beta-carotene supplements.[64]

Well-designed clinical trials and observational studies are needed to determine the short-term and long-term effects of antioxidants and cancer.[65] At this time, there are no studies nor widely accepted conclusions or extrapolations regarding benefits or problems associated with integrative use of antioxidants in veterinary clinical oncology.

Omega-3 Fatty Acids

Bauer[66] presented a dose strategy for omega-3 (N-3) FAs or N-3 polyunsaturated fatty acid, most notably eicosapentaenoic acid (EPA) and docosahexaenoic acid (DHA), for various canine diseases. Activities of matrix MMPs are significantly higher in canine malignant mammary gland tumors when compared with normal tissue. N-3 FAs affect activities of MMPs and tissue inhibitors of MMPs in dogs, suggesting potential for dietary modulation of tumor metabolism in dogs.

One clinical trial evaluated the effects of N-3 FA in 32 dogs with lymphoma: treatment dogs received a diet supplemented with menhaden fish oil and arginine, whereas control dogs received an identical diet supplemented with soybean oil. Increasing serum DHA concentration was associated with longer disease-free intervals and survival times in dogs with stage III lymphoma treated with doxorubicin.[66,67] In another study, supplementation with N-3 FA did not affect doxorubicin pharmacokinetics in 23 dogs with lymphoma.[68]

In a randomized, double-blind, placebo-controlled clinical study, 12 dogs with nasal malignant carcinomas were given dietary menhaden oil (DHA and EPA) or soybean oil (control) before radiation therapy (RT). Blood levels of DHA, EPA, insulin, glucose, lactic acid, and MMPs 2 and 9; resting energy expenditure; and inflammatory eicosanoids from nasal biopsies were measured throughout RT. The dogs fed menhaden oil had significantly higher plasma concentrations of DHA (increased by 500%) and EPA (200%), lower tissue inflammatory eicosanoids, and decreased resting energy expenditure (by 20%) compared with controls. Increased plasma DHA was significantly associated (P<.05) with decreased plasma lactic acid and MMPs. This study suggests EPA and DHA may reduce some detrimental inflammatory eicosanoids and metabolic consequences of RT.[69]

Probiotics

Current evidence demonstrates probiotic's role in modulating gut microbiota, improving gut physicochemical conditions, and reducing oxidative stress. Probiotics also inhibit tumor progression, produce anticancer compounds, and modulate the host immune response.[70,71] Evidence strongly suggests NK cells are the antitumor effector cells involved, and NK cell activity correlates with the observed antitumor effect of probiotics in mice. Dendritic cells (DC) are responsible for the recruitment and mobilization of NK cells; therefore, it may be inferred that DCs are most likely to be the acting interphase point.[72]

A large meta-analysis of probiotic use in human gastrointestinal cancer and RT to the abdominal region for cervical, ovarian, prostate, sigmoid, or colorectal cancer showed a beneficial effect.[73,74] Probiotics can improve the gut mucosal barrier by altering fecal microbes and decrease complications in humans undergoing surgery for colorectal cancer[75,76] by reducing the rate of postoperative septicemia through maintenance of gut barrier integrity in patients with colorectal cancer.[77]

RCCTs have demonstrated efficacy of probiotics, such as VSL#3, *Lactobacillus casei* DN-114 001, and other formulations, in decreasing the incidence and grade of RT-induced diarrhea, which is normally found in more than 80% of patients.[73,74,78,79]

A growing body of evidence indicates that changes in gut permeability and translocation of components of the intestinal microflora play a key role in eliciting immune-mediated mechanisms that lead to chronic inflammation, autoimmunity, and neoplasia. Research using an animal model of colorectal cancer and cachexia has shown that an increase in tumor burden leading to cachexia is accompanied by increased gut barrier permeability, elevated plasma endotoxin levels, and evidence of chronic inflammation. Improvements are reported in intestinal function, in addition to weight gain and decreased inflammation, with the use of EPA, immunoglobulin isolates, and probiotics.[80]

Contraindications to probiotic use include potential harm in several populations, including patients with neutropenia or other causes of immunosuppression, intensive care unit patients, patients with central venous catheters receiving parenteral nutrition, and patients requiring administration of the probiotic via a feeding tube.[73] A review of probiotic use in critically ill human patients lists the most commonly reported adverse events: bacteremia, fungemia, and sepsis.[81] A 2-part retrospective study conducted in 2007 to 2008 characterized probiotic use, including the type of prescribing provider, choice of probiotic prescribed, indications for use, presence of potential risk factors for probiotic infection, as well as incidence of probiotic-related bloodstream infections over 8 years. The study concluded probiotic use was associated with a minimal risk of probiotic-related infection (0.2%), despite its use at a high frequency among inpatients at high theoretic risk.[82]

In an RCCT of 40 clinically ill patients randomized to receive placebo or probiotic (VSL#3) for 7 days, patients receiving the probiotic had a reduction in inflammation and improvement of clinical outcome.[80] One systematic meta-analysis of 19 trials that studied more than 2800 infants determined that enteric probiotic supplementation significantly reduced the incidence of severe necrotizing enterocolitis; it is now being considered a standard of care in pediatric medicine. There was no evidence of significant reduction of nosocomial sepsis, and no systemic infection with supplemented probiotics in this pediatric population. This recent data and a report by the European Society for Pediatric Gastroenterology concluded probiotics could be generally considered safe at least in children.[83]

No studies have been performed in veterinary oncology patients, but the same probiotic mechanisms have been suggested in the dog and cat; therefore, veterinarians should discuss these issues with clients to design personal strategies using available products, sound clinical judgment, and the best current peer-reviewed evidence.

Phytic Acid, Phytate, Myo-Inositol Hexaphosphate

Inositol hexaphosphate (IP6; phytic acid, phytate, myo-inositol hexaphosphate) is a saturated cyclic acid found naturally in bran and seeds of plants and is the principal storage form of phosphorus. Myo-inositol is the structural basis for several secondary messengers, whereas inositol serves as an important component of the structural lipids phosphatidylinositol (PI), its various phosphates, and the phosphatidylinositol phosphate.

No RCCTs of IP6 and canine and feline cancer have been published. Early in vitro research shows IP6 slows abnormal cell division and may sometimes transform tumor cells into normal cells possessing moderate anticancer activity. The most consistent and best anticancer results were obtained from a combination of IP6 and inositol. In addition to reducing cell proliferation, IP6 increases differentiation of malignant cells, often resulting in a reversion to normal phenotype. Exogenously administered IP6 is rapidly taken into the cells and dephosphorylated to lower phosphate inositol phosphates, which further interfere with signal transduction pathways and cell-cycle arrest.[84,85]

A small randomized, pilot clinical study was conducted to evaluate IP6 + inositol in patients with breast cancer treated with adjuvant therapy. Patients receiving chemotherapy, along with IP6 + inositol, did not have cytopenia (platelets and leukocytes), had a significantly better QOL ($P = .05$) and functional status ($P = .0003$), and were able to perform their daily activities.[86]

Current literature supports the use of IP6 and is revealing the antitumor mechanisms of IP6 in vivo and in vitro, especially for breast, colorectal, and prostate cancer. Myo-inositol trispyrophosphate (ITPP), a molecule that increases oxygenation of tumor cells, increases survival of mice in a model of carcinomatosis.[87] In vitro work demonstrates that ITPP treatment increases oxygen tension and blood flow in melanoma and breast cancer models.[88]

Another study evaluated the effect of IP6 extracted from rice bran on azoxymethane-induced colorectal cancer in rats. IP6 was given via drinking water for 16 weeks, which markedly suppressed the incidence of tumors compared with the control.[89] The in vivo chemopreventive efficacy of IP6 in a mouse prostate model has also been studied using anatomic and dynamic contrast-enhanced magnetic resonance imaging.[90] A metabolomics study using quantitative high-resolution H-NMR on prostate tissue extracts showed that IP6 significantly decreased glucose metabolism and membrane phospholipid synthesis, in addition to causing an increase in myo-inositol levels in the prostate. These findings show that oral IP6 supplementation blocks growth and angiogenesis in a prostate cancer model in conjunction with metabolic events involved in tumor sustenance. The results demonstrate that energy deprivation within the tumor suppresses growth and progression of prostate cancer.[90]

An in vitro study of 3 human cancer cell lines not only confirms that IP6 alone inhibits the growth of breast cancer cells but also that IP6 acts synergistically with adriamycin or tamoxifen.[91] IP6 (2 mM) strongly inhibited both growth and proliferation, decreased cell viability, and caused a strong apoptotic death of human prostate cancer cell line, PC-3; similar effects were observed in other human cancer cell lines. These findings established, for the first time, IP6 efficacy in inhibiting aberrant epidermal growth factor receptor (EGFR) or insulin-like growth factor-1 receptor pathways; this inhibition appears to promote survival signaling cascades in advanced and androgen-independent human prostatic cancer cell lines. In another study using PC-3 tumor xenograft growth in nude mice, 2% (w/v) IP6 given in drinking water inhibited tumor growth and weight by 52% to 59% ($P<.001$). Immunohistochemical analysis of xenografts showed that IP6 significantly reduced expression of molecules associated with cell survival/proliferation (ILK1, phosphorylated Akt, cyclin D1, and proliferating cell nuclear antigen) and angiogenesis (platelet endothelial cell adhesion molecule-1 or CD31, vascular endothelial growth factor, endothelial nitric oxide synthase, and hypoxia-inducible factor-1α) together with an increase in apoptotic markers (cleaved caspase-3 and poly [ADP-ribose] polymerase [PARP]). These findings suggest that, by targeting the PI3K-ILK1-Akt pathway, IP6 suppresses cell survival, proliferation, and angiogenesis and induces prostate cancer cell death, which might have translational potential in preventing and controlling the growth of advanced and aggressive prostate cancer.[92,93]

In human colon cancer cells, IP6 up-regulates basal mRNA expression of some MMPs and their tissue inhibitors and down-regulates MMP-1, MMP-2, MMP-3, and MMP-9. IP6 could be an effective antimetastatic agent.[94]

Transforming growth factor-β (TGF-β) is a multifunctional cytokine involved in the regulation of cell development, differentiation, survival, and apoptosis with activity in neoplastic cells. In a study using colon cancer cells, another anticancer role of IP6 was shown to be enhancing the expression of the TGF-β gene and its receptors at the transcriptional level.[95]

USING IM IN VETERINARY CLINICAL ONCOLOGY

There is little high-level evidence to support use of HDS and acupuncture in veterinary clinical oncology; however, it seems reasonable to make some extrapolations, especially when considering the large amount of information from in vivo and in vitro studies in other species and the prospect of translational research. Brown and Reetz[8] set a standard with their small pilot study of PSP extract from *C versicolor*. A larger RCCT comparing effectiveness of the extract to that of doxorubicin in dogs with splenic hemangiosarcoma has been initiated.[96]

Collaboration between conventional oncologists and practitioners of IM, who have knowledge, experience, and training to use HDS and acupuncture, is needed to explore the possibilities of integrative veterinary oncology using logical, science-based practices (Erin Bannink, DVM, DACVIM [oncology], Bloomfield Hills, MI, personal communication, 2013; and Steve Marsden, DVM, ND, MSOM, L.Ac, Dipl. CH, RH [AGH], Edmonton, Alberta, Canada, personal communication, 2013). Although individual herbs are discussed here, integrative practitioners more often use herbal formulas and have identified safe, reliable sources of HDS products with known content; they also know possible interactions and understand dosing to prevent adverse effects.[10,97] Veterinarians with this special training, education, and experience can be found through the organizations in **Box 1**.

ADVERSE REACTIONS: DRUG-HERB INTERACTIONS

The most common drug-herb interactions likely occur due to altered expression of the functional CYP450 isoenzymes that metabolize chemotherapeutic drugs. A change in

---

Box 1
Sources of information about using IM in patients with cancer

- College of Integrative Therapy: www.civtedu.org
- Veterinary Information Network (message boards): www.vin.com
- American College of Veterinary Nutrition: www.acvn.org
- American Holistic Veterinary Medicine Association: www.ahvma.org
- Veterinary Botanical Medical association: www.vbma.org
- American Academe of Veterinary Acupuncture: www.aava.org
- International Veterinary Acupuncture Society: www.ivas.org

P glycoprotein (P-gp), which mediates transmembrane drug transport, is also a potential source of adverse interactions. The most notable herb-drug interaction is with *Hypericum perforatum*, more commonly known as St. John's Wort (SJW), which interferes with both CYP450 isoenzymes and P-gp. Clinical implications of drug-herb interactions depend on a variety of factors, such as dose, timing of herbal intake, dosage, route of drug administration, therapeutic range, and individual variation, including differences in the patient's diet, age, health status, genetics, and metabolizing capacity.[98,99]

A total of 66 clinical pharmacokinetic interaction studies were identified for the most frequently used herbal drugs in the United States, Canada, and Europe; the clinical evidence was most robust and informative for gingko biloba (21 studies) and milk thistle/silymarin (13), and appears limited for ginseng (9), goldenseal/berberine (8), garlic (8), and echinacea (7 studies). At commonly recommended doses, none of these herbs acted as potent or moderate inhibitors or inducers of cytochrome P450 (CYP) enzymes or P-gp.[100]

The occurrence of clinical CYP3A4-mediated interactions between anticancer drugs and SJW, milk thistle, and garlic correlated with results obtained with midazolam as a predictor of pharmacokinetic interactions. Caution is warranted when combining SJW with other anticancer drugs metabolized by CYP3A4; garlic and milk thistle were presumed safe, and no recommendation could be made for ginseng. In vitro data using CYP3A4 can likely be extrapolated to clinical studies, but clinical pharmacokinetic interactions are complicated by several factors (eg, poor pharmaceutical availability, solubility, and bioavailability of HDS). Veterinary chemotherapy drugs that use the CYP3A4 enzyme include vincristine, vinblastine, and EGFR-TK inhibitors.[101]

Curcumin, quercetin, proteolytic enzymes, ginkgo, and selenium are recommended to be discontinued during RT. Certain HDS may interfere with coagulation and are a consideration in cancer surgeries, including IP6, vitamins A and E, curcumin, and ginseng. A more comprehensive list[99] of potential interactions has been compiled, and consultation with veterinarians specializing in HDS, oncology, and nutrition to obtain the most current information is recommended.

REFERENCES

1. Deng GE, Rausch SM, Jones LW, et al. Complementary therapies and integrative medicine in lung cancer: diagnosis and management of lung cancer, 3rd edition. American College of Chest Physicians evidence-based clinical practice guidelines. Chest 2013;143(Suppl 5):e420S–36S.

2. Budgin JB, Flaherty MJ. Alternative therapies in veterinary dermatology. Vet Clin North Am Small Anim Pract 2013;43:189–204.

3. Frenkel M, Abrams DI, Ladas EJ, et al. Integrating dietary supplements into cancer care. Integr Cancer Ther 2013;12:369–84.

4. Lana SE, Kogan LR, Crump KA, et al. The use of complementary and alternative therapies in dogs and cats with cancer. J Am Anim Hosp Assoc 2006; 42:361–5.

5. Roudebush P, Davenport DJ, Novotny BJ. The use of nutraceuticals in cancer therapy. Vet Clin North Am Small Anim Pract 2004;34:249–69.

6. Memon MA, Sprunger LK. Survey of colleges and schools of veterinary medicine regarding education in complementary and alternative veterinary medicine. J Am Vet Med Assoc 2011;239:619–23.

7. Dobson JM. Breed-predispositions to cancer in pedigree dogs. ISRN Vet Sci 2013;2013:941275.

8. Brown DC, Reetz J. Single agent polysaccharopeptide delays metastases and improves survival in naturally occurring hemangiosarcoma. Evid Based Complement Alternat Med 2012;2012:384301.

9. Wang X, Sun H, Zhang A, et al. Potential role of metabolomics approaches in the area of traditional Chinese medicine: as pillars of the bridge between Chinese and Western medicine. J Pharm Biomed Anal 2011;55:859–68.

10. Marsden S. Essential guide to Chinese herbal formulas: bridging science and tradition in integrative veterinary medicine. College of Integrative Veterinary Therapies, in press.

11. Hsieh TC, Wu JM. Regulation of cell cycle transition and induction of apoptosis in HL-60 leukemia cells by the combination of Coriolus versicolor and Ganoderma lucidum. Int J Mol Med 2013;32:251–7.

12. Hsieh TC, Wu P, Park S, et al. Induction of cell cycle changes and modulation of apoptogenic/anti-apoptotic and extracellular signaling regulatory protein expression by water extracts of I'm-Yunity (PSP). BMC Complement Altern Med 2006;6:30.

13. Griessmayr PC, Gauthier M, Barber LG, et al. Mushroom-derived maitake PET-fraction as single agent for the treatment of lymphoma in dogs. J Vet Intern Med 2007;21:1409–12.

14. Skorupski KA, Hammond G, Irish AM, et al. Prospective randomized clinical trial assessing the efficacy of Denamarin for prevention of CCNU-induced hepatopathy in tumor-bearing dogs. J Vet Intern Med 2011;25:838–45.

15. Deep G, Gangar SC, Rajamanickam S, et al. Angiopreventive efficacy of pure flavonolignans from milk thistle extract against prostate cancer: targeting VEGF-VEGFR signaling. PLoS One 2012;7:e34630.

16. Jamadar-Shroff V, Papich MG, Suter SE. Soy-derived isoflavones inhibit the growth of canine lymphoid cell lines. Clin Cancer Res 2009;15:1269–76.

17. McCall JL, Burich RA, Mack PC. GCP, a genistein-rich compound, inhibits proliferation and induces apoptosis in lymphoma cell lines. Leuk Res 2010;34:69–76.

18. Morello E, Martano M, Buracco P. Biology, diagnosis and treatment of canine appendicular osteosarcoma: similarities and differences with human osteosarcoma. Vet J 2011;189:268–77.

19. Krajarng A, Nilwarankoon S, Suksamrarn S, et al. Antiproliferative effect of alpha-mangostin on canine osteosarcoma cells. Res Vet Sci 2012;93:788–94.

20. Chen XW, Sneed KB, Zhou SF. Pharmacokinetic profiles of anticancer herbal medicines in humans and the clinical implications. Curr Med Chem 2011;18: 3190–210.

21. Cretu E, Trifan A, Vasincu A, et al. Plant-derived anticancer agents—curcumin in cancer prevention and treatment. Rev Med Chir Soc Med Nat Iasi 2012;116:1223–9.
22. Jiang J, Thyagarajan-Sahu A, Loganathan J, et al. BreastDefend prevents breast-to-lung cancer metastases in an orthotopic animal model of triple-negative human breast cancer. Oncol Rep 2012;28:1139–45.
23. Li-Weber M. New therapeutic aspects of flavones: the anticancer properties of Scutellaria and its main active constituents Wogonin, Baicalein and Baicalin. Cancer Treat Rev 2009;35:57–68.
24. Lin C, Tsai SC, Tseng MT, et al. AKT serine/threonine protein kinase modulates baicalin-triggered autophagy in human bladder cancer T24 cells. Int J Oncol 2013;42:993–1000.
25. Wang CZ, Calway TD, Wen XD, et al. Hydrophobic flavonoids from Scutellaria baicalensis induce colorectal cancer cell apoptosis through a mitochondrial-mediated pathway. Int J Oncol 2013;42:1018–26.
26. Chen MC, Lee CF, Huang WH, et al. Magnolol suppresses hypoxia-induced angiogenesis via inhibition of HIF-1alpha/VEGF signaling pathway in human bladder cancer cells. Biochem Pharmacol 2013;85:1278–87.
27. Sadava D, Kane SE. Silibinin reverses drug resistance in human small-cell lung carcinoma cells. Cancer Lett 2013;339:102–6.
28. Ren L, Perera C, Hemar Y. Antitumor activity of mushroom polysaccharides: a review. Food Funct 2012;3:1118–30.
29. Torkelson CJ, Sweet E, Martzen MR, et al. Phase 1 clinical trial of Trametes versicolor in women with breast cancer. ISRN Oncol 2012;2012:251632.
30. Deng G, Lin H, Seidman A, et al. A phase I/II trial of a polysaccharide extract from Grifola frondosa (Maitake mushroom) in breast cancer patients: immunological effects. J Cancer Res Clin Oncol 2009;135:1215–21.
31. Jin X, Ruiz Beguerie J, Sze DM, et al. Ganoderma lucidum (Reishi mushroom) for cancer treatment. Cochrane Database Syst Rev 2012;(6):CD007731.
32. Chang R. Bioactive polysaccharides from traditional Chinese medicine herbs as anticancer adjuvants. J Altern Complement Med 2002;8:559–65.
33. Patel S, Goyal A. Recent developments in mushrooms as anti-cancer therapeutics: a review. 3 Biotech 2012;2:1–15.
34. Youn MJ, Kim JK, Park SY, et al. Potential anticancer properties of the water extract of Inonotus [corrected] obliquus by induction of apoptosis in melanoma B16-F10 cells. J Ethnopharmacol 2009;121:221–8.
35. Bhattacharya S, Haldar PK. The triterpenoid fraction from Trichosanthes dioica root exhibits antiproliferative activity against Ehrlich ascites carcinoma in albino mice: involvement of possible antioxidant role. J Exp Ther Oncol 2012;9:281–90.
36. Vannucci L, Krizan J, Sima P, et al. Immunostimulatory properties and antitumor activities of glucans (Review). Int J Oncol 2013;43:357–64.
37. Standish LJ, Wenner CA, Sweet ES, et al. Trametes versicolor mushroom immune therapy in breast cancer. J Soc Integr Oncol 2008;6:122–8.
38. Lu W, Rosenthal DS. Acupuncture for cancer pain and related symptoms. Curr Pain Headache Rep 2013;17:321.
39. Cassileth BR, Van Zee KJ, Yeung KS, et al. Acupuncture in the treatment of upper-limb lymphedema: results of a pilot study. Cancer 2013;119:2455–61.
40. Lawenda BD, Vicini FA. Acupuncture: could an ancient therapy be the latest advance in the treatment of lymphedema? Cancer 2013;119:2362–5.
41. Chao HL, Miao SJ, Liu PF, et al. The beneficial effect of ST-36 (Zusanli) acupressure on postoperative gastrointestinal function in patients with colorectal cancer. Oncol Nurs Forum 2013;40(2):E61–8.

42. Running A, Seright T. Integrative oncology: managing cancer pain with complementary and alternative therapies. Curr Pain Headache Rep 2012;16: 325–31.
43. Lu L, Liao M, Zeng J, et al. Quality of reporting and its correlates among randomized controlled trials on acupuncture for cancer pain: application of the CONSORT 2010 Statement and STRICTA. Expert Rev Anticancer Ther 2013; 13:489–98.
44. Ezzo J, Streitberger K, Schneider A. Cochrane systematic reviews examine P6 acupuncture-point stimulation for nausea and vomiting. J Altern Complement Med 2006;12:489–95.
45. Molassiotis A. Managing cancer-related fatigue with acupuncture: is it all good news for patients? Acupunct Med 2013;31:3–4.
46. Trump DL, Muindi J, Fakih M, et al. Vitamin D compounds: clinical development as cancer therapy and prevention agents. Anticancer Res 2006;26:2551–6.
47. Rassnick KM, Muindi JR, Johnson CS, et al. In vitro and in vivo evaluation of combined calcitriol and cisplatin in dogs with spontaneously occurring tumors. Cancer Chemother Pharmacol 2008;62:881–91.
48. Rassnick KM, Muindi JR, Johnson CS, et al. Oral bioavailability of DN101, a concentrated formulation of calcitriol, in tumor-bearing dogs. Cancer Chemother Pharmacol 2011;67:165–71.
49. Malone EK, Rassnick KM, Wakshlag JJ, et al. Calcitriol (1,25-dihydroxycholecalciferol) enhances mast cell tumour chemotherapy and receptor tyrosine kinase inhibitor activity in vitro and has single-agent activity against spontaneously occurring canine mast cell tumours. Vet Comp Oncol 2010;8:209–20.
50. Kaewsakhorn T, Kisseberth WC, Capen CC, et al. Effects of calcitriol, seocalcitol, and medium-chain triglyceride on a canine transitional cell carcinoma cell line. Anticancer Res 2005;25:2689–96.
51. Konety BR, Lavelle JP, Pirtskalaishvili G, et al. Effects of vitamin D (calcitriol) on transitional cell carcinoma of the bladder in vitro and in vivo. J Urol 2001;165: 253–8.
52. Kim SH, Chen G, King AN, et al. Characterization of vitamin D receptor (VDR) in lung adenocarcinoma. Lung Cancer 2012;77:265–71.
53. Sokolowska-Wojdylo M, Lugowska-Umer H, Maciejewska-Radomska A. Oral retinoids and rexinoids in cutaneous T-cell lymphomas. Postepy Dermatol Alergol 2013;30:19–29.
54. de Mello Souza CH, Valli VE, Selting KA, et al. Immunohistochemical detection of retinoid receptors in tumors from 30 dogs diagnosed with cutaneous lymphoma. J Vet Intern Med 2010;24:1112–7.
55. Klebanoff CA, Spencer SP, Torabi-Parizi P, et al. Retinoic acid controls the homeostasis of pre-cDC-derived splenic and intestinal dendritic cells. J Exp Med 2013;210:1961–76.
56. Bengtsson AM, Jönsson G, Magnusson C, et al. The cysteinyl leukotriene 2 receptor contributes to all-trans retinoic acid-induced differentiation of colon cancer cells. BMC Cancer 2013;13:336.
57. Waters DJ, Shen S, Cooley DM, et al. Effects of dietary selenium supplementation on DNA damage and apoptosis in canine prostate. J Natl Cancer Inst 2003; 95:237–41.
58. Waters DJ, Shen S, Kengeri SS, et al. Prostatic response to supranutritional selenium supplementation: comparison of the target tissue potency of selenomethionine vs. selenium-yeast on markers of prostatic homeostasis. Nutrients 2012; 4:1650–63.

59. Ben-Arye E, Polliack A, Schiff E, et al. Advising patients on the use of non-herbal nutritional supplements during cancer therapy: a need for doctor-patient communication. J Pain Symptom Manage 2013;46:887–96.

60. Husain K, Francois RA, Yamauchi T, et al. Vitamin E delta-tocotrienol augments the antitumor activity of gemcitabine and suppresses constitutive NF-kappaB activation in pancreatic cancer. Mol Cancer Ther 2011;10:2363–72.

61. Block KI, Koch AC, Mead MN, et al. Impact of antioxidant supplementation on chemotherapeutic efficacy: a systematic review of the evidence from randomized controlled trials. Cancer Treat Rev 2007;33:407–18.

62. Block KI, Koch AC, Mead MN, et al. Impact of antioxidant supplementation on chemotherapeutic toxicity: a systematic review of the evidence from randomized controlled trials. Int J Cancer 2008;123:1227–39.

63. Bjelakovic G, Nikolova D, Simonetti RG, et al. Systematic review: primary and secondary prevention of gastrointestinal cancers with antioxidant supplements. Aliment Pharmacol Ther 2008;28:689–703.

64. Cortes-Jofre M, Rueda JR, Corsini-Muñoz G, et al. Drugs for preventing lung cancer in healthy people. Cochrane Database Syst Rev 2012;(10):CD002141.

65. Greenlee H, Hershman DL, Jacobson JS. Use of antioxidant supplements during breast cancer treatment: a comprehensive review. Breast Cancer Res Treat 2009;115:437–52.

66. Bauer JE. Therapeutic use of fish oils in companion animals. J Am Vet Med Assoc 2011;239:1441–51.

67. Ogilvie GK, Fettman MJ, Mallinckrodt CH, et al. Effect of fish oil, arginine, and doxorubicin chemotherapy on remission and survival time for dogs with lymphoma: a double-blind, randomized placebo-controlled study. Cancer 2000; 88:1916–28.

68. Selting KA, Ogilvie GK, Gustafson DL, et al. Evaluation of the effects of dietary n-3 fatty acid supplementation on the pharmacokinetics of doxorubicin in dogs with lymphoma. Am J Vet Res 2006;67:145–51.

69. Hansen RA, Anderson C, Fettman MJ, et al. Menhaden oil administration to dogs treated with radiation for nasal tumors demonstrates lower levels of tissue eicosanoids. Nutr Res 2011;31:929–36.

70. Kahouli I, Tomaro-Duchesneau C, Prakash S. Probiotics in colorectal cancer (CRC) with emphasis on mechanisms of action and current perspectives. J Med Microbiol 2013;62(Pt 8):1107–23.

71. Orlando A, Russo F. Intestinal microbiota, probiotics and human gastrointestinal cancers. J Gastrointest Cancer 2013;44:121–31.

72. Feyisetan O, Tracey C, Hellawell GO. Probiotics, dendritic cells and bladder cancer. BJU Int 2012;109:1594–7.

73. Bazzan AJ, Newberg AB, Cho WC, et al. Diet and nutrition in cancer survivorship and palliative care. Evid Based Complement Alternat Med 2013;2013: 917647.

74. Shadad AK, Sullivan FJ, Martin JD, et al. Gastrointestinal radiation injury: prevention and treatment. World J Gastroenterol 2013;19:199–208.

75. Liu Z, Qin H, Yang Z, et al. Randomised clinical trial: the effects of perioperative probiotic treatment on barrier function and post-operative infectious complications in colorectal cancer surgery—a double-blind study. Aliment Pharmacol Ther 2011;33:50–63.

76. Zhu D, Chen X, Wu J, et al. Effect of perioperative intestinal probiotics on intestinal flora and immune function in patients with colorectal cancer. Nan Fang Yi Ke Da Xue Xue Bao 2012;32:1190–3 [in Chinese].

77. Liu ZH, Huang MJ, Zhang XW, et al. The effects of perioperative probiotic treatment on serum zonulin concentration and subsequent postoperative infectious complications after colorectal cancer surgery: a double-center and double-blind randomized clinical trial. Am J Clin Nutr 2013;97:117–26.
78. Visich KL, Yeo TP. The prophylactic use of probiotics in the prevention of radiation therapy-induced diarrhea. Clin J Oncol Nurs 2010;14:467–73.
79. Xue H, Sawyer MB, Wischmeyer PE, et al. Nutrition modulation of gastrointestinal toxicity related to cancer chemotherapy: from preclinical findings to clinical strategy. JPEN J Parenter Enteral Nutr 2011;35:74–90.
80. Ebrahimi-Mameghani M, Sanaie S, Mahmoodpoor A, et al. Effect of a probiotic preparation (VSL#3) in critically ill patients: a randomized, double-blind, placebo-controlled trial (Pilot Study). Pak J Med Sci 2013;29:490–4.
81. Theodorakopoulou M, Perros E, Giamarellos-Bourboulis EJ, et al. Controversies in the management of the critically ill: the role of probiotics. Int J Antimicrob Agents 2013;42(Suppl):S41–4.
82. Simkins J, Kaltsas A, Currie BP. Investigation of inpatient probiotic use at an academic medical center. Int J Infect Dis 2013;17:e321–4.
83. Alfaleh K, Anabrees J. Efficacy and safety of probiotics in preterm infants. J Neonatal Perinatal Med 2013;6:1–9.
84. Vucenik I, Shamsuddin AM. Cancer inhibition by inositol hexaphosphate (IP6) and inositol: from laboratory to clinic. J Nutr 2003;133(11 Suppl 1):3778s–84s.
85. Vucenik I, Shamsuddin AM. Protection against cancer by dietary IP6 and inositol. Nutr Cancer 2006;55:109–25.
86. Bacic I, Druzijanić N, Karlo R, et al. Efficacy of IP6 + inositol in the treatment of breast cancer patients receiving chemotherapy: prospective, randomized, pilot clinical study. J Exp Clin Cancer Res 2010;29:12.
87. Derbal-Wolfrom L, Pencreach E, Saandi T, et al. Increasing the oxygen load by treatment with myo-inositol trispyrophosphate reduces growth of colon cancer and modulates the intestine homeobox gene Cdx2. Oncogene 2013;32:4313–8.
88. Kieda C, El Hafny-Rahbi B, Collet G, et al. Stable tumor vessel normalization with pO(2) increase and endothelial PTEN activation by inositol trispyrophosphate brings novel tumor treatment. J Mol Med (Berl) 2013;91:883–99.
89. Shafie NH, Mohd Esa N, Ithnin H, et al. Preventive inositol hexaphosphate extracted from rice bran inhibits colorectal cancer through involvement of Wnt/beta-catenin and COX-2 pathways. Biomed Res Int 2013;2013:681027.
90. Raina K, Ravichandran K, Rajamanickam S, et al. Inositol hexaphosphate inhibits tumor growth, vascularity, and metabolism in TRAMP mice: a multiparametric magnetic resonance study. Cancer Prev Res (Phila) 2013;6:40–50.
91. Tantivejkul K, Vucenik I, Eiseman J, et al. Inositol hexaphosphate (IP6) enhances the anti-proliferative effects of adriamycin and tamoxifen in breast cancer. Breast Cancer Res Treat 2003;79:301–12.
92. Gu M, Raina K, Agarwal C, et al. Inositol hexaphosphate downregulates both constitutive and ligand-induced mitogenic and cell survival signaling, and causes caspase-mediated apoptotic death of human prostate carcinoma PC-3 cells. Mol Carcinog 2010;49:1–12.
93. Gu M, Roy S, Raina K, et al. Inositol hexaphosphate suppresses growth and induces apoptosis in prostate carcinoma cells in culture and nude mouse xenograft: PI3K-Akt pathway as potential target. Cancer Res 2009;69:9465–72.
94. Kapral M, Wawszczyk J, Jurzak M, et al. The effect of inositol hexaphosphate on the expression of selected metalloproteinases and their tissue inhibitors in IL-1beta-stimulated colon cancer cells. Int J Colorectal Dis 2012;27:1419–28.

95. Kapral M, Wawszczyk J, Hollek A, et al. Induction of the expression of genes encoding TGF-beta isoforms and their receptors by inositol hexaphosphate in human colon cancer cells. Acta Pol Pharm 2013;70:357–63.

96. University of Pennsylvania School of Veterinary Medicine. Further evaluation of the benefits of a traditional Chinese medicine supplement for dogs with splenic hemangiosarcoma. Available at: http://www.vet.upenn.edu/research/clinical-trials/vcic/penn-vet-clinical-trials/clinical-trial/further-evaluation-of-the-benefits-of-a-traditional-chinese-medicine-supplement-for-dogs-with-splenic-hemangiosarcoma. Accessed April 3, 2014.

97. Shmalberg J, Hill RC, Scott KC. Nutrient and metal analyses of Chinese herbal products marketed for veterinary use. J Anim Physiol Anim Nutr (Berl) 2013;97:305–14.

98. Pal D, Mitra AK. MDR- and CYP3A4-mediated drug–herbal interactions. Life Sci 2006;78:2131–45.

99. Noe JE. Textbook of naturopathic integrative oncology. Toronto: CCNM Press; 2012. p. 287.

100. Hermann R, von Richter O. Clinical evidence of herbal drugs as perpetrators of pharmacokinetic drug interactions. Planta Med 2012;78:1458–77.

101. Goey AK, Mooiman KD, Beijnen JH, et al. Relevance of in vitro and clinical data for predicting CYP3A4-mediated herb-drug interactions in cancer patients. Cancer Treat Rev 2013;39:773–83.

102. Jung MH, Lee SH, Ahn EM, et al. Decursin and decursinol angelate inhibit VEGF-induced angiogenesis via suppression of the VEGFR-2-signaling pathway. Carcinogenesis 2009;30:655–61.

103. Zhang J, Li L, Jiang C, et al. Anti-cancer and other bioactivities of Korean Angelica gigas Nakai (AGN) and its major pyranocoumarin compounds. Anticancer Agents Med Chem 2012;12:1239–54.

104. Zhang Y, Shaik AA, Xing C, et al. A synthetic decursin analog with increased in vivo stability suppresses androgen receptor signaling in vitro and in vivo. Invest New Drugs 2012;30(5):1820–9.

105. Yance DR Jr, Sagar SM. Targeting angiogenesis with integrative cancer therapies. Integr Cancer Ther 2006;5:9–29.

106. Weifeng T, Feng S, Xiangji L, et al. Artemisinin inhibits in vitro and in vivo invasion and metastasis of human hepatocellular carcinoma cells. Phytomedicine 2011;18:158–62.

107. Crespo-Ortiz MP, Wei MQ. Antitumor activity of artemisinin and its derivatives: from a well-known antimalarial agent to a potential anticancer drug. J Biomed Biotechnol 2012;2012:247597.

108. Chen HW, Lin IH, Chen YJ, et al. A novel infusible botanically-derived drug, PG2, for cancer-related fatigue: a phase II double-blind, randomized placebo-controlled study. Clin Invest Med 2012;35:E1–11.

109. Huang C, Xu D, Xia Q, et al. Reversal of P-glycoprotein-mediated multidrug resistance of human hepatic cancer cells by Astragaloside II. J Pharm Pharmacol 2012;64:1741–50.

110. Zhang D, Zhuang Y, Pan S, et al. Investigation of effects and mechanisms of total flavonoids of Astragalus and calycosin on human erythroleukemia cells. Oxid Med Cell Longev 2012;2012:209843.

111. Guo L, Bai SP, Zhao L, et al. Astragalus polysaccharide injection integrated with vinorelbine and cisplatin for patients with advanced non-small cell lung cancer: effects on quality of life and survival. Med Oncol 2012;29:1656–62.

112. Liu Y, Jia Z, Dong L, et al. A randomized pilot study of atractylenolide I on gastric cancer cachexia patients. Evid Based Complement Alternat Med 2008;5:337–44.

113. Plengsuriyakarn T, Viyanant V, Eursitthichai V, et al. Anticancer activities against cholangiocarcinoma, toxicity and pharmacological activities of Thai medicinal plants in animal models. BMC Complement Altern Med 2012;12:23.
114. Zhao W, Entschladen F, Liu H, et al. Boswellic acid acetate induces differentiation and apoptosis in highly metastatic melanoma and fibrosarcoma cells. Cancer Detect Prev 2003;27:67–75.
115. Kirste S, Treier M, Wehrle SJ, et al. Boswellia serrata acts on cerebral edema in patients irradiated for brain tumors: a prospective, randomized, placebo-controlled, double-blind pilot trial. Cancer 2011;117:3788–95.
116. Lu XL, He SX, Ren MD, et al. Chemopreventive effect of saikosaponin-d on diethylinitrosamine-induced hepatocarcinogenesis: involvement of CCAAT/enhancer binding protein beta and cyclooxygenase-2. Mol Med Rep 2012;5:637–44.
117. Cheng YL, Lee SC, Lin SZ, et al. Anti-proliferative activity of Bupleurum scrozonerifolium in A549 human lung cancer cells in vitro and in vivo. Cancer Lett 2005;222:183–93.
118. Wang Q, Zheng XL, Yang L, et al. Reactive oxygen species-mediated apoptosis contributes to chemosensitization effect of saikosaponins on cisplatin-induced cytotoxicity in cancer cells. J Exp Clin Cancer Res 2010;29:159.
119. Roh JS, Han JY, Kim JH, et al. Inhibitory effects of active compounds isolated from safflower (Carthamus tinctorius L.) seeds for melanogenesis. Biol Pharm Bull 2004;27:1976–8.
120. Zhao PW, Wang DW, Niu JZ, et al. Evaluation on phytoestrogen effects of ten kinds of Chinese medicine including Flos carthami. Zhongguo Zhong Yao Za Zhi 2007;32:436–9 [in Chinese].
121. Shi X, Ruan D, Wang Y, et al. Anti-tumor activity of safflower polysaccharide (SPS) and effect on cytotoxicity of CTL cells, NK cells of T739 lung cancer in mice. Zhongguo Zhong Yao Za Zhi 2010;35:215–8 [in Chinese].
122. Eom KS, Kim HJ, So HS, et al. Berberine-induced apoptosis in human glioblastoma T98G cells is mediated by endoplasmic reticulum stress accompanying reactive oxygen species and mitochondrial dysfunction. Biol Pharm Bull 2010;33:1644–9.
123. Manoharan S, Sindhu G, Vinothkumar V, et al. Berberine prevents 7,12-dimethylbenz[a]anthracene-induced hamster buccal pouch carcinogenesis: a biochemical approach. Eur J Cancer Prev 2012;21:182–92.
124. Singh IP, Mahajan S. Berberine and its derivatives: a patent review (2009-2012). Expert Opin Ther Pat 2013;23:215–31.
125. Zanotto-Filho A, Grandhi BK, Thakkar A, et al. The curry spice curcumin selectively inhibits cancer cells growth in vitro and in preclinical model of glioblastoma. J Nutr Biochem 2012;23:591–601.
126. Sutaria D, Grandhi BK, Thakkar A, et al. Chemoprevention of pancreatic cancer using solid-lipid nanoparticulate delivery of a novel aspirin, curcumin and sulforaphane drug combination regimen. Int J Oncol 2012;41:2260–8.
127. Shehzad A, Lee YS. Molecular mechanisms of curcumin action: signal transduction. Biofactors 2013;39:27–36.
128. Liu D, Chen Z. The effect of curcumin on breast cancer cells. J Breast Cancer 2013;16:133–7.
129. Qiao Q, Jiang Y, Li G. Inhibition of the PI3K/AKT-NF-kappaB pathway with curcumin enhanced radiation-induced apoptosis in human Burkitt's lymphoma. J Pharmacol Sci 2013;121:247–56.

130. Wei X, Zhou D, Wang H, et al. Effects of pyridine analogs of curcumin on growth, apoptosis and NF-kappaB activity in prostate cancer PC-3 cells. Anticancer Res 2013;33:1343–50.

131. Feng X, Zhang L, Zhu H. Comparative anticancer and antioxidant activities of different ingredients of Ginkgo biloba extract (EGb 761). Planta Med 2009;75:792–6.

132. Richardson MA. Biopharmacologic and herbal therapies for cancer: research update from NCCAM. J Nutr 2001;131(Suppl 11):3037s–40s.

133. Jia L, Zhao Y, Liang XJ. Current evaluation of the millennium phytomedicine-ginseng (II): Collected chemical entities, modern pharmacology, and clinical applications emanated from traditional Chinese medicine. Curr Med Chem 2009; 16:2924–42.

134. Li B, Zhao J, Wang CZ, et al. Ginsenoside Rh2 induces apoptosis and paraptosis-like cell death in colorectal cancer cells through activation of p53. Cancer Lett 2011;301:185–92.

135. Park D, Bae DK, Jeon JH, et al. Immunopotentiation and antitumor effects of a ginsenoside Rg(3)-fortified red ginseng preparation in mice bearing H460 lung cancer cells. Environ Toxicol Pharmacol 2011;31:397–405.

136. Park B, Lee YM, Kim JS, et al. Neutral sphingomyelinase 2 modulates cytotoxic effects of protopanaxadiol on different human cancer cells. BMC Complement Altern Med 2013;13:194.

137. Marx WM, Teleni L, McCarthy AL, et al. Ginger (Zingiber officinale) and chemotherapy-induced nausea and vomiting: a systematic literature review. Nutr Rev 2013;71:245–54.

138. Lee J, Oh H. Ginger as an antiemetic modality for chemotherapy-induced nausea and vomiting: a systematic review and meta-analysis. Oncol Nurs Forum 2013;40:163–70.

139. Liu Y, Whelan RJ, Pattnaik BR, et al. Terpenoids from Zingiber officinale (Ginger) induce apoptosis in endometrial cancer cells through the activation of p53. PLoS One 2012;7(12):e53178.

140. Hu R, Zhou P, Peng YB, et al. 6-Shogaol induces apoptosis in human hepatocellular carcinoma cells and exhibits anti-tumor activity in vivo through endoplasmic reticulum stress. PLoS One 2012;7(6):e39664.

141. In LL, Arshad NM, Ibrahim H, et al. 1′-Acetoxychavicol acetate inhibits growth of human oral carcinoma xenograft in mice and potentiates cisplatin effect via proinflammatory microenvironment alterations. BMC Complement Altern Med 2012;12:179.

142. Sung B, Prasad S, Yadav VR, et al. Cancer cell signaling pathways targeted by spice-derived nutraceuticals. Nutr Cancer 2012;64:173–97.

143. Wang KL, Hsia SM, Chan CJ, et al. Inhibitory effects of isoliquiritigenin on the migration and invasion of human breast cancer cells. Expert Opin Ther Targets 2013;17:337–49.

144. Chilampalli C, Guillermo R, Zhang X, et al. Effects of magnolol on UVB-induced skin cancer development in mice and its possible mechanism of action. BMC Cancer 2011;11:456.

145. Singh T, Prasad R, Katiyar SK. Inhibition of class I histone deacetylases in non-small cell lung cancer by honokiol leads to suppression of cancer cell growth and induction of cell death in vitro and in vivo. Epigenetics 2013;8:54–65.

146. Vaid M, Sharma SD, Katiyar SK. Honokiol, a phytochemical from the Magnolia plant, inhibits photocarcinogenesis by targeting UVB-induced inflammatory mediators and cell cycle regulators: development of topical formulation. Carcinogenesis 2010;31:2004–11.

147. Kauntz H, Bousserouel S, Gossé F, et al. Silibinin triggers apoptotic signaling pathways and autophagic survival response in human colon adenocarcinoma cells and their derived metastatic cells. Apoptosis 2011;16:1042–53.
148. Kauntz H, Bousserouel S, Gossé F, et al. The flavonolignan silibinin potentiates TRAIL-induced apoptosis in human colon adenocarcinoma and in derived TRAIL-resistant metastatic cells. Apoptosis 2012;17:797–809.
149. Cho JK, Park JW, Song SC. Injectable and biodegradable poly(organophospha-zene) gel containing silibinin: its physicochemical properties and anticancer activity. J Pharm Sci 2012;101:2382–91.
150. Piao BK, Wang YX, Xie GR, et al. Impact of complementary mistletoe extract treatment on quality of life in breast, ovarian and non-small cell lung cancer patients. A prospective randomized controlled clinical trial. Anticancer Res 2004;24:303–9.
151. Maletzki C, Linnebacher M, Savai R, et al. Mistletoe lectin has a shiga toxin-like structure and should be combined with other Toll-like receptor ligands in cancer therapy. Cancer Immunol Immunother 2013;62:1283–92.
152. Yan Z, Zhu ZL, Wang HQ, et al. Pharmacokinetics of panaxatrol disuccinate sodium, a novel anti-cancer drug from Panax notoginseng, in healthy volunteers and patients with advanced solid tumors. Acta Pharmacol Sin 2010;31:1515–22.
153. Yan Z, Yang R, Jiang Y, et al. Induction of apoptosis in human promyelocytic leukemia HL60 cells by panaxynol and panaxydol. Molecules 2011;16:5561–73.
154. Wang ZJ, Song L, Guo LC, et al. Induction of differentiation by panaxydol in human hepatocarcinoma SMMC-7721 cells via cAMP and MAP kinase dependent mechanism. Yakugaku Zasshi 2011;131:993–1000.
155. Wang W, Zhang X, Qin JJ, et al. Natural product ginsenoside 25-OCH3-PPD inhibits breast cancer growth and metastasis through down-regulating MDM2. PLoS One 2012;7(7):e41586.
156. Chao JC, Chiang SW, Wang CC, et al. Hot water-extracted Lycium barbarum and Rehmannia glutinosa inhibit proliferation and induce apoptosis of hepatocellular carcinoma cells. World J Gastroenterol 2006;12:4478–84.
157. Son YO, Lee SA, Kim SS, et al. Acteoside inhibits melanogenesis in B16F10 cells through ERK activation and tyrosinase down-regulation. J Pharm Pharmacol 2011;63:1309–19.
158. Huang Y, Hu J, Zheng J, et al. Down-regulation of the PI3K/Akt signaling pathway and induction of apoptosis in CA46 Burkitt lymphoma cells by baicalin. J Exp Clin Cancer Res 2012;31:48.
159. Huang ST, Wang CY, Yang RC, et al. Wogonin, an active compound in Scutellaria baicalensis, induces apoptosis and reduces telomerase activity in the HL-60 leukemia cells. Phytomedicine 2010;17:47–54.
160. Liu S, Ma Z, Cai H, et al. Inhibitory effect of baicalein on IL-6-mediated signaling cascades in human myeloma cells. Eur J Haematol 2010;84:137–44.
161. Park KI, Park HS, Kang SR, et al. Korean Scutellaria baicalensis water extract inhibits cell cycle G1/S transition by suppressing cyclin D1 expression and matrix-metalloproteinase-2 activity in human lung cancer cells. J Ethnopharmacol 2011;133:634–41.
162. Xu XF, Cai BL, Guan SM, et al. Baicalin induces human mucoepidermoid carcinoma Mc3 cells apoptosis in vitro and in vivo. Invest New Drugs 2011;29:637–45.

Role of Surgery in Multimodal Cancer Therapy for Small Animals

 CrossMark

Sarah Boston, DVM, DVSc[a],*, Ralph A. Henderson Jr, DVM, MS[b]

KEYWORDS

• Surgical oncology • Resection • Adjuvant therapy • Chemotherapy • Radiation

KEY POINTS

• Surgery is an essential component of the diagnosis and treatment of cancer in small animals.
• The method of biopsy and of tumor removal can have a significant impact on outcome.
• Once a diagnosis is made and the patient is staged, the dose of surgery and timing of adjuvant therapies should be planned by the oncology team before initiating any therapies.
• It is critical that the surgical oncologist has a good understanding of the impact of chemotherapy and radiation on surgical patients and that the surgical site is treated appropriately if postoperative radiation is part of the multimodal plan.

Surgery is the mainstay in the diagnosis and treatment of most solid tumors in small animals. It can be used as sole therapy in some situations, but often is used in concert with adjuvant therapies such as chemotherapy and radiation. It is critical that the surgical oncologist has a good understanding of surgical oncology principles; cancer biology; and the roles of surgery, radiation, chemotherapy, and novel therapies in treating neoplasia. The methods of biopsy for diagnosis and staging are often at least in part the responsibility of the surgeon and can have a considerable impact on patient outcome. A qualified surgeon has the technical ability to perform complicated procedures; however, the skill of selecting the best procedure that compliments an integrated plan for cancer treatment is what differentiates a general surgeon from a surgical oncologist.

Disclosures: None.
[a] Department of Small Animal Clinical Sciences, College of Veterinary Medicine, University of Florida, 2015 Southwest 16th Avenue, PO Box 100116, Gainesville, FL 32610, USA;
[b] Veterinary Surgical Consulting, 1021 Moores Mill Road, Auburn, AL 36830, USA
* Corresponding author.
E-mail address: sboston@ufl.edu

Vet Clin Small Anim 44 (2014) 855–870
http://dx.doi.org/10.1016/j.cvsm.2014.05.008
0195-5616/14/$ – see front matter © 2014 Elsevier Inc. All rights reserved.

PREOPERATIVE EVALUATION

The initial task of the surgeon is to obtain a diagnosis. The first step in this process often involves a fine-needle aspirate, and, although this is a recommended step in getting a diagnosis, cytology is prone to inaccuracy because the pathologist receives a small sample of cells lacking in vivo orientation. Before a major surgical procedure, a histologic diagnosis is recommended. The suitable type of biopsy may be a Tru-Cut, incisional, or excisional biopsy, and the decision making behind which biopsy technique is most appropriate varies with the size, location, and presumptive or cytologic diagnosis of the mass. Regardless of the method of biopsy, the biopsy tract must be resected with the definitive resection and the biopsy incision should be oriented to facilitate this. In addition, the tissue planes surrounding the mass must not be disrupted by the biopsy procedure. A solid mass should not be removed without knowledge of the tumor type (an unplanned excision). Unplanned excisions are often associated with an excision that is larger than is necessary to remove the gross disease only, but not large enough to remove all microscopic disease. In addition, the unplanned excision has the potential to disrupt the surrounding fascia and may be oriented in a manner that makes reexcision challenging.

Staging for local and distant extent of disease is critical before surgical planning. The staging performed depends on the suspected or confirmed tumor type. Three-dimensional imaging is useful in screening for occult metastatic disease, although availability and costs can limit its use. It is difficult to generalize about the appropriate method for staging solid tumors, but computed tomography (CT) scan of the mass, thorax, and possibly the abdomen for local and distant staging and incisional biopsy of the mass after evaluating the images is a highly efficient way to obtain a lot of information about the extent of disease and a definitive diagnosis. Surgical staging may also involve surgical removal or biopsy of local lymph nodes, which may be combined with initial diagnostics or definitive resection. Various aspects of initial staging can be performed using minimally invasive techniques, which may reduce overall morbidity associated with tumor staging.

SURGICAL TREATMENT

Once the histologic diagnosis, grade, and extent of disease are known, a surgical plan can be made based on the predicted biological behavior of the disease and the owner's goals for therapy. A comprehensive plan that takes into account the need for and the timing of adjuvant therapy should be developed before a surgical intervention. The goals of surgery may be palliative or curative.

The difference between palliative and curative intent treatment is not always clear, and these goals can be thought of as a continuum, rather than as absolutes. However, in general terms, palliative-intent surgery is intended to achieve cytoreduction of the tumor to relieve clinical signs, improve the patient's quality of life, and/or to allow adjuvant therapies to have the greatest impact on residual disease. Often palliative surgery is performed when local and/or metastatic control is not possible. Palliative surgery may be intralesional, in which gross disease remains, or preferably marginal, in which all macroscopic tumor burden is removed, if possible. Another goal of palliative surgery is a tension-free closure that heals with minimal complications. These goals should be balanced when deciding between an intralesional versus a marginal excision.

Surgery may also play a role in palliation when metastasectomy is performed. Guidelines for pulmonary metastasectomy have been reported in human oncology. CT scan is used to monitor metastatic lung nodules; the number of nodules, disease-free interval, and tumor doubling time are important factors in decision making.[1–4] In veterinary oncology, pulmonary metastasectomy for the management of canine osteosarcoma was reported by O'Brien and colleagues[5] in 1994. Disease-free interval between local control of primary appendicular osteosarcoma and the appearance of lung metastasis and the number of nodules were prognostic. Liptak and colleagues[6] also reported pulmonary metastasectomy in 4 dogs with osteosarcoma for the management of hypertrophic osteopathy. Because these studies were performed using radiography to evaluate the lungs for metastasis, reassessment of these recommendations using CT scan would be useful. Another change in veterinary surgery since the publication of this article is the increasing use of thoracoscopy to remove lung lesions, which may be more palatable to some owners compared with thoracotomy.[7,8] In veterinary medicine, metastasectomy is routinely performed in cases of canine anal sac adenocarcinoma, for which cytoreduction by extirpation of the iliolumbar node bed along with resection of the primary anal sac adenocarcinoma has been shown to lead to prolonged survival times with adjuvant chemotherapy.[9,10] Further, the presence of lymph node involvement has not been shown to have a negative impact on survival time if the nodes are removed as part of the surgical treatment.[10]

SURGICAL ONCOLOGY PRINCIPLES

Curative intent or definitive surgical therapy has the goal of local control of the tumor. Some tumor cells have the ability to break free from the parent mass and infiltrate the surrounding tissues, establishing microscopic satellite neoplasms. Often these leader cells cannot be seen grossly, but presumably they are there with certain types of tumors because of the high rates of local recurrence with marginal excision and because of evidence of infiltrative cells at histologic margins when a wide excision is not performed. The existence of these infiltrative cells has led to the dogma that malignant tumors must be resected with a wide or radical excision to achieve local control. A wide excision involves 2-cm to 3-cm radial margins and a fascial layer deep to the tumor, which is best planned with three-dimensional imaging. Fascia is used as the deep margin because it serves as a barrier to most tumor cells, which tend to infiltrate to, but not through, the fascia under the tumor (a notorious exception to this is the sarcoma cells of feline injection sites, for which even larger margins of 5 cm radially and 2 fascial planes deep are recommended[11]). The fascial plane that is used depends on tumor location; it may be true fascia overlying a muscle if it is possible to remove it from the muscle as a contiguous sheet. The fascial layer may also be the muscle, bone, or the chest wall, depending on tumor location. The tumor pseudocapsule, subcutaneous tissue, and fat cannot be considered a fascial plane and cannot be used as a deep layer in curative intent tumor resection. One uncommon exception to this guideline is in obese patients, for whom metric margins of 3 cm can be taken around the mass, including the deep layer. In these cases, a large metric margin may be sufficient as a deep margin. When the surgical margins are reported by the pathologist, the radial margins should be reported as a metric margin and the deep layer should be reported with the quality of the margin and not the metric distance. Radical excision involves the resection of an anatomic compartment in cases in which curative intent surgery is the goal, but cannot be achieved with a wide resection.

Intraoperative principles of surgical oncology are followed to minimize the risk of potential neoplastic cell contamination of areas beyond the tumor bed. Surgical instruments and gloves should be changed when shifting sites or masses during biopsy or excision. Within 1 tumor resection, different gloves and instruments must be used when harvesting a skin graft or flap for reconstruction. When dirty margins are anticipated during marginal resection, changing gloves and instruments for closure is unlikely to result in a different outcome. When a wide or radical resection is performed and clean margins are anticipated, changing gloves and instruments for closure is also unlikely to change the outcome, even with dirty margins. If the tumor capsule is inadvertently entered during resection, the site should be closed with suture and lavaged with copious amounts of saline. Gloves and instruments should be changed and the surgery should continue with larger margins than originally planned. This unfortunate occurrence is rare and can be prevented by careful surgical planning using three-dimensional imaging.

Drains should be used judiciously in surgical oncology. Prevention of seroma formation is important because seroma formation can lead to contamination of the tissues surrounding the tumor bed with neoplastic cells if there is a marginal excision and/or dirty margins and it can be difficult to accurately treat this area with reexcision or radiation therapy. The use of gravity-depending Penrose drains should be avoided in general because they require that the drain is tunneled from the tumor bed to a distant ventral site. With dirty margins, contamination of the drain tract results in the need either to resect this tract or treat it with radiation, which can prove difficult. A Penrose drain can be used if the egress site can be optimized. However, closed-suction drains have several distinct advantages, the most important of which is that the exit point can be adjacent to the primary incision and that this drain site can easily be included in a future resection or radiation field if necessary.

ROLE OF THE HISTOPATHOLOGIST

It is essential that critical information is transferred from surgeon to pathologist and back to the surgeon. The history, gross description, and inking of surgical margins assist with accuracy of the histopathologic diagnosis and margin assessment. Painting the entire specimen with tissue ink results in random margin assessment. Margins of concern should be inked with a different color and the pathologist should be alerted. Otherwise, the cranial, caudal, ventral, and dorsal margins should be inked, as well as the deep margin. The deep margin should be inked directly under the main mass because this is the location where the cells are most likely to have invaded the underlying fascia. The pathologist's report should include a complete description that would allow another pathologist to report a diagnosis, grade, and margin assessment without seeing the slides.[12] The surgeon should read the entire report, paying particular attention to the number of mitotic figures, amount of necrosis, invasion into lymphatic and blood vessels, and degree of differentiation.

A disadvantage of histopathology as a method of margin assessment is the delays caused by tissue processing. During surgery, frozen section is uncommonly performed in veterinary medicine to assess margins, largely because of lack of availability and lack of training of veterinary pathologists in these techniques. These procedures also result in the loss of diagnostic material for fixed histopathology. A new technique in human surgical oncology that may be feasible in veterinary medicine is imprint cytology, or touch-prep evaluation, of surgical margins during surgery. The sensitivity and specificity of intraoperative imprint cytology compared with definitive margin evaluation in human patients having breast cancer lumpectomy has been reported to be 97% to 100% and 99% to 100%, respectively.[13,14] Although not yet evaluated in veterinary surgical oncology, advantages include a rapid procedure that does not require additional equipment or training if cytologist support is readily available. Further, the diagnostic material from the main specimen is not lost. Another novel technique for the real-time evaluation of the surgical margin is the intraoperative assessment of the tumor bed for residual neoplastic cells using a fluorescent probe and imaging device. In the only report of this technique in dogs with soft tissue sarcoma, the histologic surgical margins correlated with the intraoperative results of the imaging device in 9 out of 10 cases.[15]

CHEMOTHERAPY AND SURGERY

In general, chemotherapy is indicated as adjuvant therapy in solid tumors in which the potential for metastatic spread is greater than 50%. The most common scenario in veterinary medicine when surgery and chemotherapy are both part of the treatment plan is that surgery is performed first and adjuvant chemotherapy is administered 10 to 14 days later, usually at the time of suture removal. The advantages of this approach are that it limits the potential for chemotherapy to have an effect on wound healing or to compound the effects of surgical complications such as infection. The other advantages of removing the tumor before chemotherapy is that surgery is performed sooner, which may improve quality of life in some patients, and that this allows time for the histopathology to be reported, which may be helpful in developing the overall plan for the patient going forward.

Most chemotherapeutic agents do not influence surgical wound healing; however, high-dose corticosteroid administration delays the inflammatory phase of wound healing and nonabsorbable or slowly absorbable sutures should be used. Skin suture removal should be delayed until healing is complete. Other information on the effect of chemotherapy on wound healing is sparse. In rat models, there is evidence that doxorubicin administration has an effect on wound strength when it is administered within 7 days before surgery. This effect seems to be mitigated when the drug is administered 14 days or more before surgery.[16–18] Another study using a wound model in rats also showed a significant decrease in wound strength when doxorubicin was administered up to 21 days after a wound was created, with this effect being mitigated when chemotherapy was delayed until 28 days after wounding, indicating that postoperative adjuvant chemotherapy may also have an impact on surgical wound strength.

If neoadjuvant chemotherapy is being considered, another practical reason to postpone surgery for a period after chemotherapy administration is the nadir (the lowest value of the blood cell count [neutrophils and/or platelets] after chemotherapy administration). It varies depending on the chemotherapy drug administered, but is usually 7 to 21 days after administration. Surgeons must be aware of the chemotherapy protocol that their surgical patients are receiving and the nadir of each of these chemotherapeutic agents, which is important for planning the timing of surgery and also when managing any postoperative complications while a patient is on chemotherapy. Before taking a patient having chemotherapy to surgery, a complete blood count (CBC) must be performed to ensure that it is safe to do so. If the cell counts are too low, supportive care should be given as needed and the CBC should be monitored until recovery.

The use of neoadjuvant chemotherapy is rarely reported in veterinary medicine. Although chemotherapy is not considered to be most effective against bulky disease, neoadjuvant chemotherapy been reported in human oncology to facilitate resection and often limb salvage in cases of osteosarcoma and soft tissue sarcoma.[19,20] In veterinary medicine, neoadjuvant chemotherapy has been considered to facilitate resection in a small number of reports. Large mast cell tumors in dogs can present a surgical challenge and neoadjuvant prednisone has been reported to enable resection; however, the recurrence rate in this study was 23.8%,[21] which suggests that neoadjuvant prednisone facilitates a marginal resection, but may not allow complete removal of the mass. This strategy might be most effective when cytoreduction is the goal of surgery. Prednisone is likely to decrease the size of the tumor caused by inflammation, but does not change the infiltrative pattern of the malignant mast cells within the tumor bed. Neoadjuvant chemotherapy with toceranib and cytotoxic chemotherapy have been anecdotally reported for mast cell tumors in dogs, but no data on its efficacy exist.

Neoadjuvant doxorubicin has been reported in dogs with nonresectable subcutaneous hemangiosarcoma and, in 4 of 18 cases, the tumor response led to complete tumor resection. However, these patients did not have an improvement in survival time.[22] Neoadjuvant carboplatin has also been reported in dogs with appendicular osteosarcoma, with no difference in survival time between dogs given neoadjuvant versus adjuvant chemotherapy and limb amputation.[23] Neoadjuvant chemotherapy's most useful application may be in cases of solid tumors that are not resectable and in which a partial response may facilitate marginal or complete resection.

Nonsteroidal antiinflammatory drugs and low-dose, continuous chemotherapy, also known as metronomic chemotherapy, have recently been used in veterinary oncology to treat a variety of neoplasms through modulation of T-lymphocyte populations and antiangiogenesis. Small molecule inhibitors (tyrosine kinase inhibitors) are also being used with increasing frequency. Because of the antiangiogenic effects of both classes of medication, especially with the small molecule inhibitors, the risk of adverse effects on wound healing is significant. Animals receiving single-agent toceranib or imatinib therapy should have the drug withdrawn for a minimum of 1 week before performing surgery. Continuing the drug rest for a minimum of 2 weeks during healing seems prudent because most neovascularization is attenuating in wound healing after 2 weeks. Complex, difficult, and high-risk wounds should probably be rested from these drugs until healing is satisfactory as judged by the surgeon.

COMBINING RADIOTHERAPY WITH SURGERY

Radiation can be combined with surgery as a second local treatment of the management of neoplasms.[24] Radiation therapy (radiotherapy) can be administered systemically, internally, or externally. High-energy photon teletherapy (x-rays and gamma-rays) passes through tissues regardless of tissue density. In contrast, radiation with electron teletherapy can be delivered to a partial thickness of a body part, thereby sparing critical deeper structures. Photon and electron teletherapy can be combined. Partial-thickness penetration is useful for intraoperative dosing of radiation so that a high locally targeted dose is delivered once during surgery. After surgery, high-energy photons (fully penetrating) are administered to boost the dose to the target while minimizing the dose to normal tissue.

Teletherapy is usually delivered from linear accelerators (LINACs) or cobalt sources. Both can deliver state-of-the-art x-ray or gamma radiation, respectively, but LINACs are more versatile because the source can be moved and the beam can be manipulated by a variety of collimators. Radiation oncologists plan the treatments and work with radiation physicists and technologists for radiation delivery. Multiple factors are considered, including neoplasm size/density, location, nearby risk structures, local tissue health, depth of dose needed, total dose needed, and risk of early and late treatment effects.

Stereotactic radiosurgery (SRS) is a treatment variant usually reserved for small neoplasms (<3 cm) with precise margins. SRS is typically performed in the brain or spinal cord in lieu of surgery. Precise administration of a single high radiation dose is the defining feature of SRS. Stereotactic body radiation treatment (SBRT)/stereotactic radiation treatment (SRT) is similar and the term is applied to non–central nervous system sites. SBRT delivers higher total doses through use of multiple fractions, but uses fewer fractions (usually <5) than conventional radiotherapy. The primary advantage of SRS/SBRT/SRT is that a high dose of radiation can be administered to a precise target, with a sharp decrease in the radiation dose to the adjacent tissues.

Although usually administered through the skin, radiation also can be delivered during surgery with intraoperative radiation therapy.[25] The surgeon exposes and isolates the target field with a sterile, transparent overdrape. A single high radiotherapy dose is delivered to the exposed tissue. The wound is closed and after surgery and additional radiation treatments are delivered with external doses. The advent of stereotactic radiation treatment has decreased the need for intraoperative radiation therapy, because the tissues can be spared from the radiation field through precise administration, rather than by surgical isolation.

Deciding whether radiotherapy should follow surgery is not difficult. Because of their complimentary nature as local treatments, sequential application of surgery and radiation should be considered whenever the application of either modality alone seems unlikely to effect a cure. Because both surgeon and radiation therapist must be aware of diagnosis and grade as well as volume, location, stage, and anticipated behavior of a neoplasm, the sequencing plan should be discussed before either treatment is initiated. The discussion is important because although these treatments are complimentary, they also can complicate one another.

Surgery alone is most effective as a treatment of neoplasms that are well defined and located in body regions where normal tissue can be removed with and encapsulate the neoplasm, the so-called margin, and still have sufficient tissue for local reconstruction. If the surgeon thinks that the neoplasm can be completely removed, extirpative surgery with curative intent should be considered as the frontline treatment. The few exceptions to this axiom are neoplasms that are highly sensitive to radiation (or chemotherapy) and if the cosmetic or functional values are judged to exceed the increased cost of radiotherapy. If the surgeon thinks that a clean surgical margin is not possible, an adjunct treatment with radiation should be considered. Radiation treatment is most effective as a treatment when the neoplastic cells are of smaller volume, well oxygenated, dividing rather than resting, and where surrounding normal cells in the margin can be sufficiently protected. The surgeon's role is to understand that large neoplasms have increased populations of resting, hypoxic, and dying cells that are resistant to irradiation, so cytoreductive surgery that removes the less susceptible cells is beneficial to successful irradiation of the remnant neoplasm. If this approach is taken, the goal is cytoreduction and a tension-free closure, with a flat, simple scar that will heal readily so that radiotherapy can be initiated as soon as possible.

RESPONSE OF NORMAL TISSUE TO RADIATION

Because radiation induces change in normal tissue, adversely affects wound healing, and complicates surgical procedures in previously operated tissues, it is important to begin with a brief review of the effects of radiation on normal tissue. More details are available in targeted reviews.[26–29] Cellular injury results from random ionizing events and random cell death. Ionization produces accumulation of intracellular free radicals that, with direct radiation injury, may induce critical disruption of DNA or organelles. With irreparable damage, cells typically die within 4 cell divisions.[30] Depending on the particular cell population, cell death may occur during mitosis, interphase, or subclinical apoptosis, and some cells may leave senescence through differentiation.

The science behind radiotherapy, radiobiology, is substantial and sophisticated. However, like surgery, clinical radiotherapy has also included much clinical trial and experience derived from individual patient variation. In addition, much of the science continues to be extrapolated from unfractionated (single, large) total doses,[31,32] whereas clinical radiation is usually administered in multiple fractions. The responses of normal tissues to irradiation are described in operational terms as acute, consequential, and late effects rather than more modern mechanistic terms that better describe the underlying cellular and molecular events.[33]

Acute radiation effects develop within hours to days of irradiation and are explained by injury to a population of cells undergoing rapid turnover. When acute responses become clinical, their significance is more related to the individual's response to tissue irradiation than to the dose. Clinical signs result from the loss of a sufficient number of cells or functional units such as when irradiated epithelium experiences normal exfoliative loss, failure of sufficient cellular replacement, and the consequences of bacterial invasion. Depending on the particular cell population, cell death may occur during mitosis, interphase, or subclinical apoptosis, and some cells may leave senescence through differentiation.

Clinical experience with tissue undergoing irradiation mandates that the tissues be examined daily. Irradiated tissues become progressively inflamed and less able to regenerate during the course of being irradiated. The response of the patient to inflammation is often self-mutilation and this must be prevented. Such behavior should be detected early and topical medicaments, antiinflammatory medication, and physical barriers should be applied to protect the tissue. Once wounded, irradiated tissue healing is slowed and remains suppressed while irradiation continues and for an interval thereafter. Because stem cells tend to be resistant to irradiation, they are the source of healing in irradiated tissues. The rate of healing depends on the supportive care provided to the tissues, the health of stem cells, and the native tissue turnover.

Late radiation effects develop months to years after irradiation. Late effects tend to occur in tissues with a slower rate of turnover, such as neural tissue, fat, muscle, liver, kidney, bone, and cells with slower turnover adjacent to rapidly dividing cells, such as the intestine. The mechanisms of late effect are not thoroughly explained, but are understood in terms of the cells as a microcommunity, interrelating through cytokines, chemokines, growth factors, and other signaling molecules, which is beyond the scope of this article. Of high significance to the surgeon is the role of the vascular endothelium. Vascular endothelium lies somewhere between rapidly dividing and slowly dividing cells. To a certain extent, the dose to all tissues is limited by the dose that might induce ischemia through vascular irradiation. Damage to vasculature causes leakage, fibrin deposition, collagen production, and fibrosis; however, it is more complex than vascular leakage with cellular responses such as mast cell chymase and matrix metalloproteinase-1 (MMP1).[34] Injury to the vasculature mimics other forms of wounding and the tissues respond in a similar manner with thrombosis, induction of inflammatory cytokines, growth factors, leukocyte migration, and endothelial budding and regeneration; however, the sequence of inflammation to fibrosis results in normal tissue loss or dysfunction. Some tissues may be partially rescued after radiation injury. Laboratory-manipulated human lipoaspirates (fat) infused into irradiated (single dose of 45 Gy) subcutaneous tissues of wild-type friend lukemia virus B (FVB) mice experienced a downregulation of transforming growth factor beta/SMAD gene family member 3 (TGF-β/SMAD3) (profibrosis) response and decreased collagen production.[35] Placement of breast implants in human beings after mastectomy and radiation have been considered a surgery of higher risk for failure. Autografting of fat into the subcutis permitted successful alloplastic implant reconstruction.[36] Such microenvironmental restructuring alteration is only one of many avenues being evaluated to modulate radiation injury. However, cytokine and growth factor–driven tissue repair might also provide harmful stimuli if neoplastic tissue remains in treated tissues.

Consequential late effects are acute reactions that fail to heal completely and persist into the late period. For instance, irradiated stem cells may be unable to differentiate fully because of constitutive or microenvironmental alterations.[37] Such primary lesions add to the overall damage.[38] There seems to be an increase in occurrence and risk for consequential late effects because of well-established syndromes like radiation recall, in which inflammation recurs in irradiated tissue when certain chemotherapeutic and other drugs are administered systemically.[39] Aggressive new combined treatment regimens, especially with antiangiogenic chemotherapeutics, small molecule therapy, and targeted therapy pose additional threat for consequential effects. As if the relationship of radiation and normal tissue were not complicated enough, the neoplasm and its satellites produce cellular mediators that can modify the local tissue environments and compromise normal tissue response or recovery. In addition, although uncommon in veterinary patients, radiation can induce oncogenesis.

SURGERY OF TISSUE TO BE IRRADIATED

Surgery interposed before or after tissue irradiation further increases the complexity of radiation treatment by introducing wounded tissue into the equation. Normal wound healing is a highly ordered sequence of vasocellular migration and proliferation events that are modulated by growth factors, cytokines, interleukins, proteinases, and other factors. Repetitive wound irradiation disrupts this progression resulting in repetitive inflammatory stimuli, cell injury, and imbalance of wound modulators even though irradiation promotes many of the same factors found in normal wound healing. The veterinary literature is numerically weak on the subject of healing of irradiated wounds.[24] One longitudinal clinical study showed that skin flaps prepared in 26 dogs that were subsequently irradiated experienced complication in 20 for which 6 required reoperation and 4 remained unresolved.[40] Flaps that were planned as a part of the initial tumor resection and reconstruction had a higher success rate than those designed to correct a problem or failure of radiotherapy.

There is an adage that states that tissue often heals in spite of the surgical technique. This adage is not true for most irradiated wounds. Besides inducing damage to the normalcy of tissue, radiation further delays healing by multiple mechanisms such as inducing endothelial apoptosis and reducing basic fibroblast growth factor (bFGF)[41] and MMP1.[42] Surgery for tissues that are to receive irradiation requires optimal operative attention that begins with the discussion between the surgeon and radiation oncologist as to the probable type of radiation treatment required. The depth and composition of the wound determine whether and which radiation treatments might be considered. The wound should be prepared to optimize the radiation oncologist's ability to treat. If the depth of tissue to be irradiated is greater than 3 cm (or if electrons are not available), photon radiotherapy is required and different surgical care is used. The optimum surgical wound for photon radiation results in a zone of injury well demarcated by judicious placement of steel or titanium vascular clips or skin staples[43] and a wound well supported by sutures. The most important consideration for the radiation oncologist is adequate targeting of the neoplastic wound remnant (bed) and a sufficient margin of surrounding tissue. After a surgical wound has been closed, the internal changes are impossible for the radiation oncologist to imagine. How deep? How much undermining? How much shifting of tissue has taken place secondary to wound tension and closure? From the outside, the wound is the center of the lesion and although this view is refined for planning by intravenously contrasted, cross-sectional imaging, the surgeon can further assist by placing internal fiduciary markers (**Fig. 1**).

In body sites where full penetration by photon radiotherapy risks inducing lethal secondary effects, electron radiation is considered as an alternative treatment. Shallow electron fields are more demanding for the surgeon because, if not properly prepared, electron therapy may have to be abandoned because of probable failure. For best (uniform) dosimetry, the optimum surgical wound for electron radiation results in a wound bed of uniform thickness, flat surface, compact symmetry, absence of osseous or metallic obstructions, and is well supported with suture.

Wound geometry influences dosimetry and electron delivery. In flat, compact surgical wounds, electrons are easier to deliver because dose distribution loses uniformity if the wound differs in depth or if the body falls away over a curve. As particles, electrons are impeded by mass and the denser the mass the more rapid the dose reduction. Even soft tissue inhomogeneity can adversely influence dose distribution, but, more importantly, the presence of dense tissue, bone, or metallic implants can attenuate or block electrons and spare neoplastic cells. Electron radiation is not used in fields where neoplasm may be blocked by bone or implants. When appropriate, the surgeon should remove potentially obstructing bone and limit hemostatic methods to ligature and electrocoagulation, never metallic clips.

Conventional excision techniques result in wounds that are less compact than necessary. For example, most linear incisions must be approximately 1.5 times the length of a subcutaneous mass for adequate primary skin retraction and visualized excision. A linear excision that incorporates skin lengthens during closure because the curved edges are straightened. The length of these excisions can be reconfigured by using a curvilinear incision; usually of S shape (**Fig. 2**), which results in an incision of similar length for access, but that is more constrained for a rectangular field for irradiation.

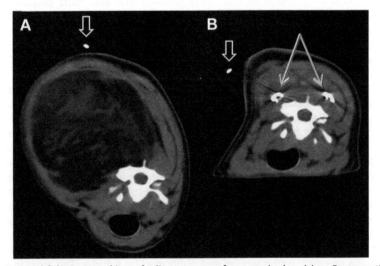

Fig. 1. Internal fiduciary marking of a liposarcoma after marginal excision. Preoperative (*A*) and postoperative (*B*) corresponding cervical spine CT images. Note the external fiduciary markers (*open arrows*) and internal staples (*thin arrows*) to assist the radiotherapist in treatment planning. Multiple staples were placed, particularly at the depth of the wound to assist planning to protect the cervical spinal cord.

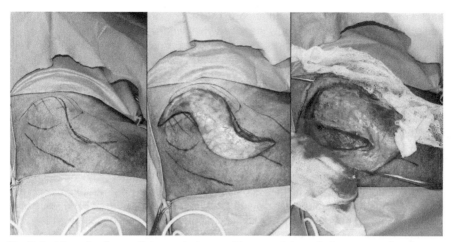

Fig. 2. Incision plan for partial scapulectomy with potential need of postoperative electron irradiation. Sketch of anatomic and disease structure overlain by S-shaped incision plan (*left*). S-curved incision (*middle*) permits reflection of flaps that improve access to the deeper structures (*right*). The plan achieves visualization with a compact wound. This closure does not extend over the dorsal body curvature and is absent angular flaps as with a T incision.

Wounds that are to receive radiation should be closed with the simplest tension-free technique. Wound tissue must be supported for longer than normal healing and remodeling periods so permanent or long-lasting monofilament sutures are recommended. The placement of drains is preferable to tissues separated by seroma. If a drain is placed, the egress sites must be able to be incorporated into the irradiated field. If drains are required for wound care, healing is delayed and radiation should also be delayed until tissue union is progressing. Anatomic layered closure including an intradermal layer is optimal. The skin may be sutured or stapled; however, if support of the wound throughout irradiation is desirable and wound closure will remain, a small gauge continuous suture will accommodate both photon and electron therapy.

Depending on the nature of the species, area wounded, tissues injured, and thoroughness of apposition on closure, radiation may commence immediately after surgery or be delayed. Cats seem to be more resistant to the acute effects of tissue irradiation than dogs. Simple wounds survive irradiation better than complexly reconstructed wounds. Well-apposed linear wounds in cats may begin to receive radiation as early as the same day of surgery. Nonlinear wounds are allowed to heal for 2 to 3 weeks before initiating irradiation. Although well-apposed linear wounds of dogs seem to heal satisfactorily, it is common to permit healing to continue for a minimum of 2 weeks before proceeding to irradiation. Wounds with complex angles and flaps are delayed for up to 4 weeks.

OPERATING IN IRRADIATED TISSUE

Operating in irradiated tissue is occasionally planned, but more often it is required to manage nonhealing ulcers and reoperation for recurrence of neoplasia. Useful veterinary reports are few. Retrospective studies occasionally remark on radiation toxicity, but less commonly relate surgery complicated by radiotherapy. In a retrospective study of nasal neoplasms receiving radiotherapy or radiotherapy followed by exenteration, the investigators concluded that radiotherapy may increase the risk of surgical complications. Dogs receiving radiotherapy followed by exenteration had increased relative risk for nonhealing nasocutaneous fistula, osteomyelitis, osteonecrosis, and rhinitis, but they had a significantly longer survival time.[44]

Fibroplasia that occurs in irradiated tissue obliterates natural tissue planes and, surgically, the tissues are sticky, requiring sharp dissection or electrosection similar to removal of an inflamed lymph node or anal sac. Nerves are of similar texture to connective tissue and vessels are hidden so dissection in irradiated tissue is less precise and is accompanied by higher risks for injury to collateral near-field structures. When possible, surgery should be delayed until healing has progressed well into the remodeling period, beyond the natural production of elastin in the wounded area (usually beyond 1 month from healing), which results in the best possible tissue conditions. Preoperative planning for critical areas could be preceded by contrast imaging (magnetic resonance, CT, ultrasound). Surgery should be conducted with patience and finesse. The core surgical principles of dissection (primary wound retraction, accurate section, hemostasis, traction with countertraction, and avoidance of blind undercutting dissection) do not differ from those of conventional surgical oncology and reconstruction. The surgeon similarly cannot rely as much on the forgiveness of the healing processes in irradiated tissues. Even free vascularized tissue grafts have a higher complication rate when applied to irradiated tissue.[45] Free-graft survival is mostly unknown in veterinary medicine at present but was shown to be improved in a subsequent study by the topical application of vascular endothelial growth factor (VEGF).[46]

Should an entire irradiated tissue field be removed? Under most considerations, if complete surgical removal is possible, surgery should have already been performed as the frontline therapy. However, there are circumstances in which radiotherapy is elected by the clinician or owner rather than surgery as the frontline treatment, because of a likely successful response, and when presurgical radiation improves the probability of successful multimodal therapy. This strategy has been used for feline injection site sarcoma, with preoperative radiation followed by resection.[47] There is not a clear rule as to which approach is better in feline injection site sarcoma: preoperative radiation followed by surgery, or surgery followed by radiation.[48] Each case needs to be considered individually. However, the ability to achieve clean margins of resection seems to be the most significant factor in successful treatment of this disease.[11,47]

In instances in which radiation has been performed before surgery, such as failed nasal planum radiotherapy for squamous cell carcinoma, clinical experience has

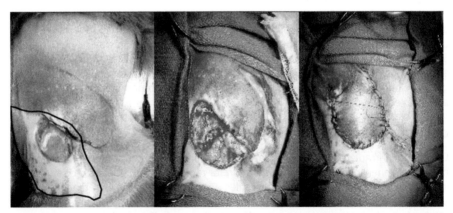

Fig. 3. Random rotation flap to repair radiation ulcer excision. Radiation site outlined (*left*). Excision of ulcer and flap prepared from adjacent nonirradiated tissue (*center*). Completed flap with minimal rotation torque of base and tension-free closure (*right*).

resulted in successful excision and healing. When addressing reoperation of irradiated tissue, the practical steps to consider should therefore include the aforementioned core principles and tissue flaps introduced from adjacent tissues with less radiation-induced fibrosis (**Fig. 3**). Because tissue vascularity may be compromised, tension should be minimized, flap bases emboldened, and rotation lessened. When using advancement of V-shaped tissues a rounded V tip is more likely to survive, but clinical experience suggests that complex, multi-incision wounds are at higher risk.

SUMMARY

Surgery is a critical component in the treatment of most solid tumors in small animals. Surgery is increasingly being combined with adjuvant therapies such as chemotherapy and radiation and therefore surgeons who are treating cancer must have a good understanding of surgical oncology principles, cancer biology, and the roles and potential positive and negative interactions of surgery, radiation, and chemotherapy. The sequencing plan for these modalities should be determined before any form of treatment is initiated. The first task of the surgeon is to achieve a histologic diagnosis through incisional biopsy and to stage the patient. This information can then be used to develop an integrated plan for therapy that takes into account the treatment goals as well as the best modalities for achieving local and distant disease control. Local control involves surgery and/or radiation and control of systemic spread involves adjuvant chemotherapy. During surgical resection with curative intent, surgical oncology principles must be applied to ensure complete en bloc resection of the tumor without contamination of the tumor bed.

The surgical oncologist must have a working knowledge of the chemotherapy agents with which their patients are being treated and the effect that these treatments have on both the ability of tissues to heal and the effect on the blood cell counts, especially at the nadir. In general, an interval of 2 weeks should be allowed between surgery and chemotherapy or vice versa to avoid a negative interaction of these modalities. If this is not possible, particular attention should be paid to the patient's white blood cell and platelet count and care should be taken to allow for potential delayed healing. It is also important that the surgeon is aware of the considerations of operating in tissues before and after irradiation. Considerations that the surgeon should make if a mass is being resected marginally, with a plan to follow with adjuvant radiation, include the placement of metallic fiduciary markers at the internal limits of the surgical wound. Planning for electron radiotherapy is assisted if the surgeon composes a flat, compact wound of uniform thickness that contains no bone or metal that would block electrons. Wounds to be irradiated should be apposed by layers, tension free, and sutured with nonabsorbable or slowly absorbable suture. Simple, well-apposed wounds may be irradiated immediately, but wounds that are under tension, that required drains, or that required complex reconstruction should be rested until near the end of the proliferation phase of wound healing (beyond week 3). Radiation causes fibrosis in normal tissues, obliterating normal fascial separations. Surgery of irradiated tissue is hazardous because dissection must be sharp, vascular and neural structure is obscured, and vascular support for healing is already compromised. A good working knowledge of the surgical management of tumors with and without the addition of neoadjuvant or adjuvant therapies is essential to successful multimodal therapy for cancer in small animals.

REFERENCES

1. Gilson S. Principles of surgery for palliation and treatment of metastasis. Clin Tech Small Anim Pract 1998;13:65–9.

2. Virgo KS, Naunheim KS, Johnson FE. Preoperative workup and postoperative surveillance for patients undergoing pulmonary metastasectomy. Thorac Surg Clin 2006;16:125–31.
3. Detterbeck FC, Grodzki T, Gleeson F, et al. Imaging requirements in the practice of pulmonary metastasectomy. J Thorac Oncol 2010;5:S134–139.
4. Nichols FC. Pulmonary metastasectomy. Thorac Surg Clin 2012;22:91–9.
5. O'Brien MG, Straw RC, Withrow SJ, et al. Resection of pulmonary metastases in canine osteosarcoma: 36 cases (1983-1992). Vet Surg 1993;22:105–9.
6. Liptak JM, Monnet E, Dernell WS, et al. Pulmonary metastatectomy in the management of four dogs with hypertrophic osteopathy. Vet Comp Onc 2004;2:1–12.
7. Mayhew PD, Dunn M, Berent A. Surgical views: thoracoscopy: common techniques in small animals. Compend Contin Educ Vet 2013;35:E1.
8. Mayhew PD, Hunt GB, Steffey MA, et al. Evaluation of short-term outcome after lung lobectomy for resection of primary lung tumors via video-assisted thoracoscopic surgery or open thoracotomy in medium- to large-breed dogs. J Am Vet Med Assoc 2013;243:681–8.
9. Hobson HP, Brown MR, Rogers KS. Surgery of metastatic anal sac adenocarcinoma in five dogs. Vet Surg 2006;35:267–70.
10. Emms SG. Anal sac tumours of the dog and their response to cytoreductive surgery and chemotherapy. Aust Vet J 2005;83:340–3.
11. Phelps HA, Kuntz CA, Milner RJ, et al. Radical excision with five-centimeter margins for treatment of feline injection-site sarcomas: 91 cases (1998-2002). J Am Vet Med Assoc 2011;239:97–106.
12. Kamstock DA, Ehrhart EJ, Getzy DM, et al. Recommended guidelines for submission, trimming, margin evaluation, and reporting of tumor biopsy specimens in veterinary surgical pathology. Vet Pathol 2011;48:19–31.
13. Bakhshandeh M, Tutuncuoglu SO, Fischer G, et al. Use of imprint cytology for assessment of surgical margins in lumpectomy specimens of breast cancer patients. Diagn Cytopathol 2007;35:656–9.
14. Klimberg VS, Westbrook KC, Korourian S. Use of touch preps for diagnosis and evaluation of surgical margins in breast cancer. Ann Surg Oncol 1998;5:220–6.
15. Eward WC, Mito JK, Eward CA, et al. A novel imaging system permits real-time in vivo tumor bed assessment after resection of naturally occurring sarcomas in dogs. Clin Orthop Relat Res 2013;471:834–42.
16. Mullen BM, Mattox DE, Von Hoff DD, et al. The effect of preoperative adriamycin and dihydroxyanthracenedione on wound healing. Laryngoscope 1981;91:1436–43.
17. Khoo DB. The effect of chemotherapy on soft tissue and bone healing in the rabbit model. Ann Acad Med Singap 1992;21(2):217–21.
18. Devereux DF, Thibault L, Boretos J, et al. The quantitative and qualitative impairment of wound healing by adriamycin. Cancer 1979;43:932–8.
19. Bacci G, Longhi A, Versari M, et al. Prognostic factors for osteosarcoma of the extremity treated with neoadjuvant chemotherapy: 15-year experience in 789 patients treated at a single institution. Cancer 2006;106:1154–61.
20. O'Donnell PW, Manivel JC, Cheng EY, et al. Chemotherapy influences the pseudocapsule composition in soft tissue sarcomas. Clin Orthop Relat Res 2014;472(3):849–55.
21. Stanclift RM, Gilson SD. Evaluation of neoadjuvant prednisone administration and surgical excision in treatment of cutaneous mast cell tumors in dogs. J Am Vet Med Assoc 2008;232:53–62.

22. Wiley JL, Rook KA, Clifford CA, et al. Efficacy of doxorubicin-based chemotherapy for non-resectable canine subcutaneous haemangiosarcoma. Vet Comp Oncol 2010;8:221–33.
23. Phillips B, Powers BE, Dernell WS, et al. Use of single-agent carboplatin as adjuvant or neoadjuvant therapy in conjunction with amputation for appendicular osteosarcoma in dogs. J Am Anim Hosp Assoc 2009;45:33–8.
24. McLeod D, Thrall D. The combination of surgery and radiation in the treatment of cancer: a review. Vet Surg 1989;18:1–6.
25. Boston SE, Duerr F, Bacon N, et al. Intraoperative radiation for limb sparing of the distal aspect of the radius without transcarpal plating in 5 dogs. Vet Surg 2007; 36:314–23.
26. Dormand E, Banwell PE, Goodacre TE. Radiotherapy and wound healing. Int Wound J 2005;2:112–27.
27. Gieringer M, Gosepath J, Naim R. Radiotherapy and wound healing: principles, management and prospects (review). Oncol Rep 2011;26:299–307.
28. Haubner F, Ohmann E, Pohl F. Wound healing after radiation therapy: review of the literature. Radiat Oncol 2012;7:162–70.
29. Stone HB, Coleman CN, Anscher MS, et al. Effects of radiation on normal tissue: consequences and mechanisms. Lancet Oncol 2003;4:529–36.
30. Thompson LH, Suit HD. Proliferation kinetics of x-irradiated mouse L cells studied with time-lapse photography. Int J Radiat Biol 1969;15:347–62.
31. Hall EJ. Dose-response relationships for model normal tissues. In: Radiobiology for the radiologist. 5th edition. Philadelphia: Lippincott Williams & Wilkins; 2000. p. 316–7.
32. Tadjalli H, Evans G, Gurlek A, et al. Skin graft survival after external beam irradiation. Plast Reconstr Surg 1999;103:1902.
33. Denham JW, Hauer-Jensen M, Peters LJ. Is it time for a new formalism to categorize normal tissue radiation injury? Int J Radiat Oncol Biol Phys 2001;50:1105–6.
34. Riekki R, Harvima IT, Jukkola A, et al. The production of collagen and the activity of mast cell-chymase increases in human skin after irradiation therapy. Exp Dermatol 2004;13:364–71.
35. Allen RJ, Scharf C, Phuong D, et al. Does fat grafting improve radiation skin damage? 26th Annual Meeting Northeastern Society of Plastic Surgeons. Available at: www.nesps.org/abstracts/2009/24.cgi. Accessed December 26, 2013.
36. Salgarillo M, Visconti G, Farello E. Autologous fat graft in radiated tissue prior to alloplastic reconstruction. Aesthetic Plast Surg 2009;34:5–10.
37. Monje ML, Mizumatsu S, Fike JR, et al. Irradiation induces neural precursor-cell dysfunction. Nat Med 2002;8:955–62.
38. Dorr W, Hendry JH. Consequential late effects in normal tissues. Radiother Oncol 2001;61:223–31.
39. Vujovic O. Radiation recall dermatitis with azithromycin. Curr Oncol 2010;17: 119–21.
40. Seguin B, McDonald D, Kent MS, et al. Tolerance of cutaneous or mucosal flaps placed into a radiation therapy field. Vet Surg 2005;34:214–22.
41. Hom DB, Unger GM, Pernell KJ, et al. Improving surgical wound healing wit bFGF after radiation. Laryngoscope 2005;115:412–22.
42. Gu Q, Wang D, Gao Y, et al. Expression of MMP1 in surgical and radiation-impaired wound healing and its effects on the healing processes. J Environ Pathol Toxicol Oncol 2002;21:71–8.
43. McEntee MC, Steffey M, Dykes NL. Use of surgical hemoclips in radiation treatment planning. Vet Radiol Ultrasound 2008;49:395–9.

44. Adams WM, Bjorling DE, McAnulty JF, et al. Outcome of accelerated radiotherapy alone or accelerated radiotherapy followed by exenteration of the nasal cavity in dogs with intranasal neoplasia: 53 cases (1990-2002). J Am Vet Med Assoc 2005; 227:936–41.
45. Schultze-Mosgau S, Grabenbauer GG, Radespiel-Troger M. Vascularization in the transition area between free grafted soft tissues and pre-irradiated graft bed tissues following preoperative radiotherapy in the head and neck region. Head Neck 2002;24:42–51.
46. Schultze-Mosgau S, Wehrhan F, Rodel F, et al. Improved vascular graft survival in an irradiated surgical site following topical application of rVEGF. Int J Radiat Oncol Biol Phys 2003;57:803–12.
47. Mayer MN, Treuil PL, LaRue SM. Radiotherapy and surgery for feline soft tissue sarcoma. Vet Radiol Ultrasound 2009;50:669–72.
48. Kobayashi T, Hauck ML, Dodge R, et al. Preoperative radiotherapy for vaccine associated sarcoma in 92 cats. Vet Radiol Ultrasound 2002;43:473–9.

Cancer Screening Tests for Small Animals

Stephanie E. Schleis, DVM

KEYWORDS

- Cancer • Companion animals • Screening tests • Diagnosis

KEY POINTS

- Biomarkers are best used in combination with other clinical findings.
- At risk breeds should be screened for the ABCB1-1Δ mutation prior to chemotherapy administration.
- No screening test should be used in isolation for diagnosis and treatment.

INTRODUCTION

Cancer is increasingly more common in our aging patient population. Increased owner expectations and advances in veterinary diagnostic capabilities have led to the development and commercial availability of several tests for the diagnosis and treatment of cancer in companion animals.

Early detection of disease may lead to more curable tumors and a less disease-debilitated patient population. However, the role of early detection in human oncology is controversial with regard to the risk-to-benefit ratio for patients. Considerations must be given to the invasiveness of procedures undergone when a screening test is positive compared with the number of patients who actually have the disease and benefit from further scrutiny. Another consideration is that, although for some cancers early detection is of survival benefit, there are others for which no evidence suggests early implementation of treatment improves the quality or quantity of life. These same discussions hold true in veterinary oncology.[1]

With the aid of objective, scientific data where available, some of the more recent cancer detection tests, albeit not an exhaustive list, are discussed herein. This article provides the reader with a basic understanding of the tests and their appropriate use for cancer diagnosis, monitoring, or predictive value for detecting cancer in a healthy patient (**Table 1**).

Disclosure: The authors have nothing to disclose.
Department of Clinical Sciences, Bailey Small Animal Teaching Hospital, Auburn University, 1010 Wire Road, Auburn, AL 36839, USA
E-mail address: ses0034@auburn.edu

Vet Clin Small Anim 44 (2014) 871–881
http://dx.doi.org/10.1016/j.cvsm.2014.05.007
0195-5616/14/$ – see front matter © 2014 Elsevier Inc. All rights reserved.

Table 1 Definitions	
Sensitivity	Proportion of patients with the disease who test positive.
Specificity	Proportion of patients without the disease who test negative.
Predictive value	Probability of disease given a particular test result. Influenced by how commonly the disease occurs in a specific population.
Biomarker	Characteristics, including substances or compounds, that are objectively measured and evaluated as indicators of normal biology, pathology, or the response to treatment.

Data from Modiano JF, Sharkey LC. A practical guide to diagnostic testing for veterinary cancer patients. 2012. Available at: www.akcchf.org/news-events/library/articles/cancerdiagnostics-1.pdf. Accessed November 1, 2013.

TESTS FOR LYMPHOMA
Veterinary Diagnostics Institute TKcanine+

This test is a recently marketed canine blood test by Veterinary Diagnostics Institute (VDI; Simi Valley, CA, USA) for the diagnostic, prognostic, and therapeutic monitoring of dogs with lymphoma and hemangiosarcoma. It employs an indirect, modified 2-step, competitive chemiluminesence immunoassay to quantify the serum level of thymidine kinase 1 (TK1), and an enzyme-linked immunosorbent assay for the quantification of serum levels of canine C-reactive protein (cCRP).

Thymidine kinase is an enzyme involved in the 1-step salvage pathway of pyrimidine synthesis. It exists in 2 forms, with TK1 located in the cytosol and TK2 located in the mitochondria.[2] TK1 is associated with cellular proliferation; its activity is greatly increased in the S phase of the cell cycle. TK1 can be measured in the serum because the enzyme can leak through the cell membrane with high levels of expression (**Fig. 1**).[2–4]

TK1 expression is limited to proliferating cells, and hematopoietic malignancies have very high cell proliferation rates.[2–5] In human oncology, serum TK1 levels provide information on prognosis and treatment efficacy in leukemia, multiple myeloma, and Hodgkin and non-Hodgkin lymphoma.[2,4,5] In veterinary species, high levels of serum TK1 compared with normal range are detected in canine lymphoma, splenic hemangiosarcoma, and feline lymphoma.[2–8] Solid tumors in dogs and humans do not show consistently increased levels precluding serum TK1 levels as a general biomarker for all cancer histologies.[3] However, it is used in humans for breast, lung, and colorectal cancer.[4] A recent study also showed increased levels of inactive TK1 in the serum of dogs with solid tumors using an immunoaffinity/Western blot assay for detection of the protein, not solely activity. The types of solid tumors included mammary tumors (n = 4), hepatic tumors (n = 2), osteosarcoma (n = 2), synovial cell sarcoma (n = 1), mastocytomas (n = 5), plasmacytoma (n = 1), fibrosarcoma (n = 1), melanoma (n = 2), histiocytic sarcoma (n = 1), lung carcinoma (n = 1), and infiltrative fibrolipoma (n = 1).[9]

Other conditions can cause an increase in the activity of serum TK1, including premalignant conditions, viral infections, and inflammatory conditions.[3] For example, TK1 was found to be significantly elevated in dogs with pyometra.[10] Based on unpublished data, minor increases in TK1 were noted concurrently with positive tests for rickettsial disease in dogs.[3] Although the specificity of TK1 as a biomarker for malignancy is high, its low-end sensitivity, especially for solid tumors, is poor owing to these other instances where TKI levels can be above the normal range.[3]

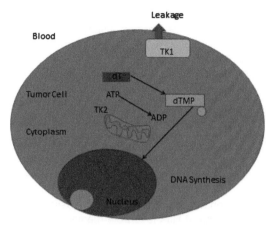

Fig. 1. Role of TK in the salvage pathway of pyrimidine synthesis. TK2 is expressed in the mitochondrion and is present during the entire cell cycle. Leakage of TK (ie, TK1) through the cell membrane reflects either the overall degree of DNA synthesis or the number of cells dying in the replicative stage. In the presence of ATP, TK1 catalyzes the conversion of deoxythymidine (dT) to deoxythymidine monophosphate (dTMP). dTMP is subsequently phosphorylated to its triphosphate analogue (dTTP) before being a substrate for DNA synthesis. (*From* von Euler H, Einarsson R, Olsson U, et al. Serum thymidine kinase activity in dogs with malignant lymphoma: a potent marker for prognosis and monitoring the disease. J Vet Intern Med 2004;18(5):696–702.)

In efforts to better the low-end sensitivity of TK1, VDI also combined with this test the detection of cCRP in serum samples.[3] cCRP is an accepted biomarker for inflammation. It is produced in the liver in response to proinflammatory cytokines as part of the acute phase response. It is an effective measure of systemic inflammation and correlates with the duration and severity of the inflammatory stimuli. However, as a biomarker it is not disease specific.[3,11–13]

Coupling biomarkers for rapid cell proliferation and inflammation has a strong relevance to the neoplastic process and malignant transformation. Chronic inflammation has been shown to predispose a patient to the development of neoplasia. The continued inflammatory state is essential in all aspects of cancer development and maintenance.[3]

In a 2013 study funded by the VDI, the resulting serum levels for each biomarker is used to create a Neoplasia Index (NI) ranging from 0 to 9. Three hundred sixty apparently healthy German shepherd dogs and golden retrievers had serum collected and analyzed for both biomarkers. The patients were followed out for a minimum of 6 months and up to 1 year after sample collection with the goal of assessing the utility of these combined biomarkers and NI to detect occult disease.[3]

During the study, 11 dogs developed malignant neoplasia and 10 developed benign tumors with an overall 3% incidence of cancer in the population. Of the 11 malignant tumors, 3 were hematopoietic and 8 were nonhematopoietic (hemangiosarcoma, abdominal sarcoma, intestinal sarcoma, anal sac adenocarcinoma, and parathyroid tumor). Results of the study showed a sensitivity of 82% and a specificity of 91% for the NI to detect occult malignant disease 6 months before the onset of clinical signs.[3]

VDI-TKcanine+ is advertised as a dual biomarker panel for dogs with suspected or confirmed cancer. Data provided by the company on their website, but not found in any peer-reviewed journals at the time of this article writing, list a patient cohort of

390 dogs with 52 cancers of various types and 22 benign neoplasms. In this population, for the diagnosis of cancer, this test had a sensitivity of 96% and specificity of 85%. A high positive sensitivity of 99% was noted when the NI was 8.0 or greater. The different varieties of cancers are not listed.[14]

Based on several other studies in dogs and humans, the ability of TK1 to function as a good biomarker for highly proliferative hematopoietic diseases such as lymphoma is known. However, caution should be used in interpreting a positive result in relation to other tumors where the biomarker has not been more thoroughly investigated. A study by Kumar and colleagues[9] demonstrated a large fraction of inactive TK1 protein in the serum of dogs with solid tumors, and an abstract by Selting and colleagues[15] in the 2013 Proceedings of the Veterinary Cancer Society may show some future significance for this biomarker combination in other tumors, but more studies need to be conducted.

The VDI also gives data on the use of TK1 as a prognostic indicator for canine lymphoma and hemangiosarcoma. It lists favorable median survival times when values are less than 30 U/L with a 50% survival probability of around 150 days. When the TK1 values are greater than 100 U/L, the median survival time is poor, at approximately 50% survival probability of 50 days. Regarding therapeutic monitoring, the company states that after successful treatment TK1/cCRP/NI should return to normal (<9 U/L, <4, and <1, respectively). Any return in elevation of these values may signify disease recurrence before the return of clinical signs.[14]

In human oncology, high serum TK1 activity has been shown to be an unfavorable prognostic factor, especially in non-Hodgkin lymphoma. The same may or may not be true in our canine patients. A 2004 study by von Euler and colleagues[2] demonstrated that TK1 activity was not significantly different from controls in dogs that had gone into remission for their lymphoma, and the TK1 levels were shown to be significantly elevated from baseline at least 3 weeks before and at the time of relapse. Dogs with initial TK1 activity of greater than 30 U/L had significantly shorter survival times. A study in 2011 assayed the TK1 activity in the serum of 73 dogs with treatment-naïve lymphoma and again after treatment. The results showed a total of 47% having an initial TK1 level greater than the reference interval; dogs with B-cell disease had a greater initial value versus those with T-cell disease. The stage of the disease did not correlate with TK1 levels (ie, higher values were not seen in higher stage disease), and TK1 activity before treatment was not associated with disease-free remission or survival. Patients with elevated levels before treatment demonstrated a decrease in levels within the normal range while responding to treatment.[7]

VDI TKFeline

VDI also offers a blood test to aid in the differentiation between feline inflammatory bowel disease and gastrointestinal lymphoma. The test only employs analysis of the levels of thymidine kinase in the serum of cats. A technical data sheet on the VDI website reports findings from a VDI study. Sixty-one cats were evaluated with 18 diagnosed with lymphoma, 12 with inflammatory bowel disease, and 31 healthy controls. The company reports significantly elevated TK1 levels in cats with lymphoma versus those with inflammatory bowel disease, or the healthy controls. It lists 78% sensitivity and 91% specificity. Although the high specificity would suggest that this test would help to rule out lymphoma, no peer-reviewed studies have been published at this time.[16]

In summary, no test can be used in a vacuum and biomarkers, especially, are best used when combined with other clinical findings. The exact role of the VDI-TKcanine+ test or VDI-TKFeline test in veterinary oncology is not fully defined. It is reasonable to pursue a more detailed diagnostic workup on patients whose values are greater than the normal ranges. The use of the test to monitor remission of lymphoma patients may also be justified; however, further work must be done before a decision can be made on the prognosis of a patient with lymphoma and response to treatment based solely on these values. Caution must be exercised when an ill patient suspected to have cancer tests negative. Further diagnostics may still be warranted, because a negative result does not exclude a malignant diagnosis. Cytotoxic treatment for patients should not be instituted based solely on a positive test. Although the return of levels greater than normal in a treated canine lymphoma patient may suggest or even support early detection of disease relapse, the role of early reinstatement of chemotherapy on overall survival has not yet been clearly defined.

Sensitest/Petscreen/Tri-Screen/Canine Lymphoma Blood Test

A joint venture between Petscreen Ltd (Nottingham, UK) and Avacta Animal Health (Wetherby, UK) has marketed the canine lymphoma blood test (cLBT). The same test can also be found under Sensitest or Tri-screen. It is marketed for the diagnosis of canine lymphoma and for the monitoring of remission status in dogs treated for lymphoma. The cLBT measures the levels of 2 acute phase proteins (APPs), cCRP and haptoglobin, in canine serum. The results of the serum levels for both biomarkers are placed in an algorithm to result in an assigned cLBT score of 0 to 5. A score of 0 for remission monitoring represents complete remission and 5 represents active disease. For the diagnosis of lymphoma, cLBT scores of 0 through 2 are negative, 2 through 3 are ambiguous, and 3 through 5 are in the positive range.[17]

A 2013 abstract by Roos and colleagues,[18] including Petscreen Limited, reported the prognostic and predictive value of the cLBT. A 92.19% sensitivity and 79.49% specificity was reported for determining detectable disease versus remission in 30 canine lymphoma patients. A cLBT of greater than 80% at day 0 was associated with a poorer prognosis, decreased time to progression (14 weeks), and overall survival time (19 weeks) compared with values of less than 80% (time to progression, 37 weeks; survival time, 59 weeks). With regard to relapse prediction, the cLBT score was found to increase significantly starting 5 weeks before clinical relapse.

Haptoglobin is an APP produced by the liver. It binds to circulating or free hemoglobin in the blood and transports free hemoglobin released from red cells back to the liver for recycling. In the dog, haptoglobin is classified as a moderately severe reacting protein induced by interleukin-6–type cytokines. Levels are elevated later in the inflammatory response and remain elevated for up to 2 weeks after the initial trigger. Haptoglobin levels can be influenced (increased) by corticosteroid administration.[13,19]

cCRP is an APP produced in the liver as part of the rapidly reacting first line of APPs induced by interleukin-1–type cytokines. Its serum levels are characterized by a dramatic increase within 4 hours after the inflammatory stimulus and rapid normalization.[19] cCRP is released as a systemic response to microbial invasion, acute inflammation, and tissue injury. cCRP concentrations have been shown to be elevated in infectious diseases such as leishmaniasis, leptospirosis, parvovirus, and ehrlichiosis. It is also elevated in inflammatory conditions such as inflammatory bowel disease, uremia, allergies, and immune-mediated, endocrine, and metabolic disease. cCRP seems to be the most sensitive APP in dogs and levels have not been shown to be altered by corticosteroid administration (**Fig. 2**).[12]

In human oncology, serum CRP concentrations have shown potential as diagnostic and prognostic markers in various neoplastic diseases, including epithelial ovarian cancer, thymic cell carcinoma, pancreatic cancer, colorectal cancer, renal cell carcinoma, and multiple myeloma.[12] Specifically, in lymphoma it has been used as a

INFLAMMATION

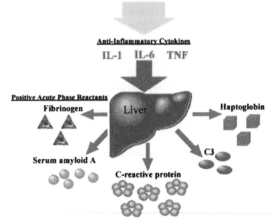

Fig. 2. Acute phase response proteins including C-reactive protein and haptoglobin. IL, interleukin; TNF, tumor necrosis factor. (*From* Hengst JM. The role of C-reactive protein in the evaluation and management of infants with suspected sepsis. Adv Neonatal Care 2003;3:3–13; with permission.)

prognostic factor and as a marker for remission and relapsed disease and correlated with stage and substage of affected patients.[12,13,19]

A 2005 study by Tecles and colleagues[13] evaluated serum concentrations of APPs haptoglobin, ceruloplasmin, serum amyloid A, and CRP in dogs. The sample cohorts included 15 healthy dogs, 12 with acute inflammation, 16 with hematologic cancer, 20 with nonhematologic cancer, and 8 with immune-mediated hemolytic anemia. There was an observed increase in concentrations of APP in all diseased individuals. However, statistical significance was only found for haptoglobin in the inflammatory and hematologic neoplasia group. Statistical significance was noted for CRP versus normal in the inflammatory, hematologic neoplasia, and immune-mediated hemolytic anemia groups. Of note, the increases in APP's for dogs with neoplasia and immune-mediated hemolytic anemia were not as elevated compared with those dogs with well-defined inflammatory processes. Also noted in this study was a strong intraindividual variation of the values.

In 2007 a study by Nielsen and colleagues[12] investigated the use of cCRP serum concentration specifically as an indicator for remission status in canine lymphoma. Serum samples were collected from 22 dogs with untreated multicentric lymphoma before starting therapy, weekly before each chemotherapy administration, and then at 1, 3, and 6 months after treatment. When patients were documented out of remission, another serum sample was collected. Results indicated a significant decrease in cCRP at the time of complete remission. Again, significant individual variation was noted between patients. In addition, the concentration of cCRP was not significantly different between substage of disease or between other remission states than complete remission, such as partial remission or even at relapse. Noted in this study, 32% of the patients had cCRP concentrations inside the reference range before treatment.

As with the Tecles study, a strong variation was noted within individuals versus between individuals. This would suggest a need for establishment of baseline levels in an individual patient if these values were to be used for monitoring the disease process in a particular patient.[12]

A study by Merlo and colleagues[11] studied the concentrations of serum cCRP in dogs with multicentric lymphoma treated with chemotherapy. Of the 20 dogs with multicentric lymphoma, only 4 had an increased serum cCRP concentration at the time of relapse. The authors suggest there may be a correlation between tumor burden and levels of cCRP. The levels increase only when there is enough tumor burden to cause tissue damage, which then incites the acute phase response. Based on this theory, cCRP alone may not function as a good early marker for return of disease in dogs before lymph node enlargement.

Most biomarkers are not optimum alone; CRP is similar. In human medicine, it is typically evaluated in a panel with other markers to assess disease. A 2007 brief communication by Mischke and colleagues[19] reported the results of a study evaluating changes in cCRP and haptoglobin in dogs with lymphatic neoplasia. The study results showed that lymphatic neoplasia was associated with significant elevations in cCRP and haptoglobin in dogs; however, it also reflected a low specificity of APPs when related to a particular disease. This observation had also been noted in 2 previous studies.

When considering the use of the cLBT, one must bear in mind the multitude of other conditions that can cause elevations in APPs. Again, results of this test should not be used alone, but rather in conjunction with other clinical findings and diagnostic/confirmatory tests. Also, if there is a plan to use the cLBT as a monitoring tool in an individual patient, a baseline level must be established for that patient at the beginning of treatment.

Polymerase Chain Reaction for Antigen Receptor Rearrangements

Polymerase chain reaction for antigen receptor rearrangements (PARR) is an objective, highly sensitive test for the detection of clonal populations of B and T lymphocytes. Specific primers are utilized to detect the unique V, D, and J gene rearrangements of the antigen-binding portion of the immunoglobulin heavy chain in B cells and the region encoding the T-cell receptor gamma in T lymphocytes. Because most lymphoid cancer is the result of clonal lymphocyte expansion, PARR allows for the differentiation between a neoplastic versus inflammatory lymphocytosis.[20]

PARR is a well-described, evaluated, and published test. It can be used in dogs and cats. In dogs, the reported sensitivity and specificity are around 90%, and in cats the sensitivity and specificity are at 89% and 80%, respectively for T-cell disease, and 60% and 70%, respectively for B-cell neoplasia.[21–23] False-negative results can occur in cases where the J or V region, which is present in the gene rearrangement in question, is not complementary to the primers in use.[20,21] The limit of detection in dogs is 1 neoplastic lymphocyte in a population of 100 heterogeneous, non-neoplastic lymphocytes.[21]

This test is offered by a variety of academic and commercial laboratories. PARR can be run on a variety of samples including blood, lymph node, bone marrow, cerebrospinal fluid, and other body fluid. Formalin-fixed samples can also be used.

PARR is a useful in determining the presence of lymphoid neoplasia, the immunophenotype, and the presence of minimal residual disease in patients receiving treatment. However, it is always important to interpret PARR results in conjunction with other findings including history, clinical signs, cytology/biopsy, flow cytometry, and immunohistochemistry, because clonal lymphocyte expansion can occur rarely in some inflammatory conditions, for example, rickettsial infections.

TESTS FOR CANINE HEMANGIOSARCOMA
VDI TKcanine+

This is the same test discussed and marketed by VDI that analyzes canine serum for levels of CRP and TK1. The use of TK1 as a biomarker for canine hemangiosarcoma was evaluated by Thamm and colleagues[6] in 2011. Researchers studied 62 dogs with hemoabdomen and 15 normal controls. The serum TK1 levels were higher in dogs with diagnosed hemangiosarcoma versus normal controls. A cutoff TK1 value of 6.55 U/L demonstrated 52% sensitivity, 93% specificity, a positive predictive value of 0.94, and a negative predictive value of 0.48 versus normal. The difference in TK1 levels between hemangiosarcoma and benign splenic disease leading to hemoabdomen was not significant. When a 2-tiered cutoff system that divided TK1 activity into low, intermediate, and high levels was used, there was improved discriminatory activity between malignant and benign splenic conditions. Very low TK1 activity (<1.55 U/L) seemed to be a good rule-out for splenic malignancy when differentiating from normal or benign splenic disease.

The role for this test in differentiating benign versus malignant splenic disease in cases of hemoabdomen or in determining prognostic significance in canine hemangiosarcoma has not been solidified. Results may support a diagnosis of hemangiosarcoma versus benign disease, but should not be used alone without histologic confirmation.

TESTS FOR CANINE TRANSITIONAL CELL CARCINOMA
Veterinary Version of the Bladder Tumor Antigen Test

A rapid latex agglutination dipstick test that allows for the qualitative detection of tumor analytes in canine urine, the veterinary version of the bladder tumor antigen test uses antibodies against a bladder tumor-associated glycoprotein complex composed of basement membrane components and immunoglobulin. This test can be easily performed in the veterinarian's office. The sensitivity of this test is reported between 85% and 90%. Specificity is reported between 41% and 86%. Of important note when using this test is that false-positive results can be observed in samples with significant glucosuria, proteinuria, pyuria, and hematuria. This confounding factor can explain the variation in specificity reported, because the test's specificity is much less in cases where the patient is showing lower urinary tract signs secondary to diseases, which can lead to urine samples containing glucose, protein, and blood.[24–27]

The veterinary version of the bladder tumor antigen test may be used as a screening test for transitional cell carcinoma of the bladder in asymptomatic patients. However, these results should not be used alone for the diagnosis and instigation of treatment for transitional cell carcinoma of the bladder. Positive results should prompt clinical evaluation with other diagnostic tests, including imaging and cytology or biopsy.

GENERAL CANCER TESTS
OncoPet RECAF

OncoPet Diagnostics and BioCurex (Los Angeles, CA, USA) offers a commercialized blood test for cancer detection in companion animals. This test detects the presence of a blood protein that is, or is similar to, the alpha-fetoprotein receptor (RECAF). Alpha-fetoprotein (AFP) is a mammalian embryo-specific and tumor-associated protein found in high amounts in the blood during fetal development and in some neoplastic conditions. It can also be present in much lesser amounts in the normal adult. AFP plays a role in cellular proliferation, differentiation, and regulation of apoptosis and immune function through signal transduction and binding to cell-surface receptors.[1,28]

AFP as a tumor-specific biomarker has long been accepted. However, it is characterized by poor sensitivity and specificity and often monitored in conjunction with other biomarkers. In addition, although AFP has been isolated in several mammalian species, its structure, mechanism of receptor binding, receptor structure, and biologic role in the embryo and carcinogenesis remains incompletely defined. The role of RECAF as a universal tumor biomarker is also not established.[1,28]

The only available data regarding the presence of RECAF in canine malignancies, the validity of the developed reagent, and any sensitivity and specificity measurements for this test is through the company. As of the writing of this article, no information with regard to this test has been published in any peer-reviewed journals.

The role of this test in the diagnosis of cancer in companion animals is not known. The results of this test should be interpreted with caution and only in conjunction with other diagnostic tests and clinical assessment.

P-glycoprotein Mutation

P-glycoprotein is a cell membrane-located pump that acts as a barrier to the distribution of substrate drugs to selected tissues. This includes restricting access through the blood–brain barrier, blood–testes barrier, and the placenta. P-glycoprotein has important excretory functions in enterocytes, biliary canalicular cells, and renal tubule epithelial cells.[29]

The gene encoding for P-glycoprotein is ABCB1 (previously named MDR1). A 4-base pair deletion mutation in this gene, referred to as the ABCB1-1Δ in canines, causes termination of protein synthesis before even 10% of the product is made. Dogs with 2 mutant alleles do not have functioning P-glycoprotein cell membrane pumps. This lack makes

Table 2
Summary

Test	Biomarker	Cancer	Use	Additional Diagnostics
VDI-TKCanine+	TK1+C-reactive protein	Lymphoma, hemangio-sarcoma	Diagnosis and monitoring of remission status	Yes
cLBT	C-reactive protein + haptoglobin	Lymphoma	Diagnosis and monitoring of remission status	Yes
PARR	Gene rearrangements of the T-cell receptor and antigen binding portion of B immunoglobulin	Lymphoid malignancy	Diagnosis through clonality status and immunophenotype	Yes
V-BTA	Tumor glycoprotein complex	Transitional carcinoma of the bladder	Screening, ruling out disease	Yes
RECAF	Alpha-fetoprotein receptor	All types	Screening	Yes
ABCB1-1Δ	Gene mutation	All types	Detection of mutation that may warrant changes in chemotherapy drugs and dosing	No

Data from Refs.[1,2,11–13,15,16,18–30]

them more susceptible to the toxicities of drugs that are substrates for this pump, including ivermectin, loperamide, doxorubicin, and vincristine, to name a few.[29,30]

There are some breeds in which the ABCB1-1Δ mutation is more prevalent. Collies, old English sheepdogs, Australian shepherds, Shetland sheepdogs, border collies, longhaired whippets, and German shepherds are just some breeds in which the mutation has been reported.[29] Individual dogs can be tested for the presence of this mutation through genotyping of blood or cheek swabs. This test has been thoroughly documented and is available through Washington State University.

Dogs with 2 mutant alleles have shown severe toxicity, even death, after receiving normal and reduced dosages of vincristine and doxorubicin.[30] These drugs are mainstays in the treatment of canine lymphoma; it is important and accepted practice to test individuals of predisposed breeds for this mutation before administering these drugs in a lymphoma protocol (**Table 2**).

REFERENCES

1. Modiano JF, Sharkey LC. A practical guide to diagnostic testing for veterinary cancer patients. 2012. Available at: www.akcchf.org/news-events/library/articles/cancerdiagnostics-1.pdf. Accessed November 1, 2013.
2. von Euler H, Einarsson R, Olsson U, et al. Serum thymidine kinase activity in dogs with malignant lymphoma: a potent marker for prognosis and monitoring the disease. J Vet Intern Med 2004;18:696–702.
3. Selting KA, Sharp CR, Ringold R, et al. Serum thymidine kinase 1 and C-reactive protein as biomarkers for screening clinically healthy dogs for occult disease. Vet Comp Oncol 2013. http://dx.doi.org/10.1111/vco.12052.
4. von Euler H, Eriksson S. Comparative aspects of the proliferation marker thymidine kinase 1 in human and canine tumor diseases. Vet Comp Oncol 2010;9(1):1–15.
5. Sharif H, von Euler H, Westberg S, et al. A sensitive and kinetically defined radiochemical assay for canine and human serum thymidine kinase 1 (TK1) to monitor canine malignant lymphoma. Vet J 2012;194:40–7.
6. Thamm DH, Kamstock DA, Sharp CR, et al. Elevated serum thymidine kinase activity in canine splenic hemangiosarcoma. Vet Comp Oncol 2011;10(4):292–302.
7. Elliott JW, Cripps P, Blackwood L. Thymidine kinase assay in canine lymphoma. Vet Comp Oncol 2011;11(1):1–13.
8. Taylor SS, Dodkin S, Papasouliotis K, et al. Serum thymidine kinase activity in clinically healthy and diseased cats: a potential biomarker for lymphoma. J Feline Med Surg 2012;15(2):142–7.
9. Kumar JK, Sharif H, Westberg S, et al. High levels of inactive thymidine kinase 1 polypeptide detected in sera from dogs with solid tumours by immunoaffinity methods: implications for in vitro diagnostics. Vet J 2013;197:854–60.
10. Sharif H, Hagman R, Wang L, et al. Elevation of serum thymidine kinase 1 in a bacterial infection: canine pyometra. Theriogenology 2013;79:17–23.
11. Merlo A, Rezende BC, Franchini ML, et al. Serum C-reactive protein concentrations in dogs with multicentric lymphoma undergoing chemotherapy. J Am Vet Med Assoc 2007;230(4):522–6.
12. Nielsen L, Toft N, Eckersall PD, et al. Serum C-reactive protein concentration as an indicator of remission status in dogs with multicentric lymphoma. J Vet Intern Med 2007;21:1231–6.
13. Tecles F, Spirane I, Bonfanti U, et al. Preliminary studies of serum acute-phase protein concentrations in hematologic and neoplastic diseases of the dog. J Vet Intern Med 2005;19:865–70.

14. Veterinary Diagnostics Institute. VDI-TKcanine+ dual biomarker panel for dogs with suspected or confirmed cancer. In: Veterinary Diagnostics Institute technical data sheet. 2012. Available at: www.vdilab.com/pdf/38_TKcanineTechSheet.pdf. Accessed November 1, 2013.

15. Selting K, Ringold R, Husbands B. Use of thymidine kinase type 1 and C-reactive protein to detect cancer in dogs [abstract]. In: Proceedings of the VCS. Minneapolis (MN): VCS; 2013. p. 58.

16. Veterinary Diagnostics Institute. VDI-TKfeline. In: Veterinary Diagnostics Institute technical data sheet. 2011. Available at: www.vdilab.com/pdf/25_TKfelineTechSheet. pdf. Accessed January 6, 2014.

17. Avacta Animal Health. Sensitest® Canine Lymphoma Blood Test (cLBT). In: Literature provided by Avacta Animal Health. Meeting of the Veterinary Cancer Society. Minneapolis, October 17–19, 2013.

18. Roos A, Jurgen T, Alexandrakis I, et al. The prognostic and predictive value of the serum C-reactive protein and haptoglobin levels in canine lymphoma [abstract]. In: Proceedings of the VCS. Minneapolis (MN): VCS; 2013. p. 59.

19. Mischke R, Waterston M, Eckersall PD. Changes in C-reactive protein and haptoglobin in dogs with lymphatic neoplasia. Vet J 2007;174:188–92.

20. Lana SE, Jackson TL, Burnett RC, et al. Utility of polymerase chain reaction for analysis of antigen receptor rearrangement in staging and predicting prognosis in dogs with lymphoma. J Vet Intern Med 2006;20:329–34.

21. Keller RL, Avery AC, Burnett RC, et al. Detection of neoplastic lymphocytes in peripheral blood of dogs with lymphoma by polymerase chain reaction for antigen receptor gene rearrangement. Vet Clin Pathol 2004;33(3):145–9.

22. Moore PF, Woo JC, Vernau W, et al. Characterization of feline T cell receptor gamma (TCRG) variable region genes for the molecular diagnosis of feline intestinal T cell lymphoma. Vet Immunol Immunopathol 2005;106:167–78.

23. Werner JA, Woo JC, Vernau W, et al. Characterization of feline immunoglobulin heavy chain variable region genes for the molecular diagnosis of B-cell neoplasia. Vet Pathol 2005;42:596–607.

24. Henry CJ, Tyler JW, McEntee MC, et al. Evaluation of a bladder tumor antigen test as a screening test for transitional cell carcinoma of the lower urinary tract in dogs. Am J Vet Res 2003;64(8):1017–20.

25. Borjesson DL, Christopher MM, Ling GV. Detection of canine transitional cell carcinoma using a bladder tumor antigen urine dipstick test. Vet Clin Pathol 1999; 28(1):33–8.

26. Billet JP, Moore AH, Holt PE. Evaluation of a bladder tumor antigen test for the diagnosis of lower urinary tract malignancies in dogs. Am J Vet Res 2002; 63(3):370–3.

27. Customer and Technical Assistance of Polymedco, Inc. V-BTATM Package Insert. 1998. Available at: www.vetbta.com/V-BTA%20Package%20Insert.html. Accessed December 1, 2013.

28. Terentiev AA, Moldogazieva NT. Alpha-fetoprotein: a renaissance. Tumour Biol 2013;34:2075–91.

29. Mealey KL, Meurs KM. Breed distribution of the ABCB1-1Δ (multidrug sensitivity) polymorphism among dogs undergoing ABCB1 genotyping. J Am Vet Med Assoc 2008;233(6):921–4.

30. Mealey KL, Northrup NC, Bentjen SA. Increased toxicity of P-glycoprotein-substrate chemotherapeutic agents in a dog with the MDR1 deletion mutation associated with ivermectin sensitivity. J Am Vet Med Assoc 2003;223(10):1453–5, 1434.

Antimicrobial Use in the Veterinary Cancer Patient

Bonnie Boudreaux, DVM, MS

KEYWORDS

- Chemotherapy • Antimicrobial • Neutropenia • Radiation • Sepsis

KEY POINTS

- Veterinarians are constantly challenged regarding prudent use of antimicrobials.
- Any patient that is displaying clinical signs around the time of the neutrophil nadir, regardless of the absolute neutrophil count, should be aggressively treated.
- Critically ill or septic patients often have special considerations that should be recognized so as to institute appropriate dosing and therapies.
- Prophylactic prescription of antimicrobials is limited to those patients considered at high risk of developing a febrile neutropenic episode after chemotherapy.
- Appropriate dosages and dosing schemes still need further work to determine the ideal treatment plan if doxycycline is to be incorporated into standard low-dose chemotherapy protocols.

ANTIMICROBIAL USE IN THE CANCER PATIENT

With the increased emergence of antimicrobial resistance in human medicine, veterinarians are constantly challenged regarding prudent use of antimicrobials. The goal of this article is to discuss the clinical indications for antimicrobial use in veterinary oncology. Areas discussed include general considerations of antimicrobial use, antimicrobials in the neutropenic patient, prophylactic antimicrobial usage, antimicrobials in radiation therapy, and antimicrobials in metronomic chemotherapy protocols.

ANTIMICROBIAL USE IN THE NEUTROPENIC PATIENT

Bone marrow suppression is the most common consequence of chemotherapeutic administration and is the dose-limiting toxicity of many chemotherapy agents.[1] Neutrophils are the cell line affected most often by chemotherapy, as they have a short life span in circulation and these cells are replenished frequently by the bone

No disclosures to report.

Veterinary Clinical Sciences, Louisiana State University, Skip Bertman Drive, Baton Rouge, LA 70803, USA

E-mail address: bbrugmann@vetmed.lsu.edu

Vet Clin Small Anim 44 (2014) 883–891

marrow.[2,3] Neutropenia frequently becomes clinically relevant approximately 7 days after administration of chemotherapeutics.[4] However, the nadir can be prolonged with the administration of certain chemotherapy drugs, including carboplatin and lomustine, which can have nadirs as late as 3 weeks after administration.[1,3,5–8]

The Veterinary Cooperative Oncology Group has established a grading scheme for neutropenia in our veterinary patients.[9] In general, most oncologists believe that if the neutrophil count is approximately 1000/μL that the body's immune system is adequate to fight an infection and the risk of infection is low.[10] However, it is critical when evaluating a patient's blood work after chemotherapy to remember that a complete blood count is simply a "snapshot in time" and there is no way to predict if the absolute neutrophil count is increasing or decreasing. Nonetheless, this number is regularly used as a set point to guide antimicrobial therapy in neutropenic chemotherapy patients as well as dose adjustments for future chemotherapy agent administrations (**Table 1**).

The greatest concern for patients that are neutropenic is for the risk of infection and subsequent sepsis. As the neutrophil count decreases, the risk of infection and septicemia increases, particularly when patients have fewer than 500 neutrophils/μL. The risk for significant side effects requiring hospitalization is less than 5%, with treatment-associated fatalities being less than 1%.[1,11]

RISK FACTORS

Two recent studies have evaluated risk factors associated with chemotherapy-induced sepsis and outcomes in veterinary patients.[12,13] Risk factors that have been identified potentially associated with chemotherapy-induced neutropenia include lower body weight, hematological tumors, chemotherapy drug used (doxorubicin/vincristine), and induction phase of chemotherapy. Additionally, factors that have been associated with a negative prognosis in dogs presenting for neutropenia episodes include hypotension, granulocyte colony-stimulating factor use, and lower rectal temperature on presentation. If any of these risk factors are identified, it may be necessary to be more aggressive with appropriate antimicrobial therapy.

FEBRILE NEUTROPENIA MANAGEMENT

Most patients with septicemia are brought to the veterinary hospital with nonspecific clinical signs and a concurrent fever. However, neutropenia by itself does not typically cause clinical signs. Therefore, any patient that is displaying clinical signs around the time of the neutrophil nadir, regardless of the absolute neutrophil count, should be aggressively treated (**Table 2**). Additionally, in some cases of severe neutropenia, the patient may have such immune dysfunction that they are unable to adequately release the necessary cytokines to produce a fever.[13] In the author's experience

Table 1					
Veterinary Cooperative Oncology Group: common terminology criteria for adverse events v1.1					
Hematologic Adverse Event	Grade 1	Grade 2	Grade 3	Grade 4	Grade 5
Neutropenia	1500/μL – lower limit of normal	1000–1499/μL	500–999/μL	<500/μL	Death

From VCOG. Veterinary Co-operative Oncology Group – common terminology criteria for adverse events (VCOG-CTCAE) following chemotherapy or biological antineoplastic therapy in dogs and cats v1.1. Vet Comp Oncol 2011. http://dx.doi.org/10.1111/j.1476-5829.2011.00283.x; with permission.

Table 2		
General guidelines for neutropenia management after chemotherapy		
Absolute Neutrophil Count	Clinical Signs	Treatment Recommendations
<3000/μL	Clinically well	Delay chemotherapy
<1000/μL	Clinically well	Delay chemotherapy, prescribe oral antimicrobials
<3000/μL	Febrile, sick	Hospitalize, parenteral antimicrobials, supportive care

and as documented by Britton and colleagues,[13] these patients are often the most critical. Patients presenting with febrile neutropenia should immediately receive intravenous broad-spectrum antimicrobials. Broad-spectrum antimicrobial coverage in the neutropenic patient should target aerobic gram-positive, gram-negative, and anaerobic bacteria.[1,3,10] For most chemotherapy patients who are in their normal home environment, the source of septicemia is bacterial translocation from their own gastrointestinal tract. Other sources or sites of infection that should be evaluated include the urinary tract, respiratory tract, and skin. Careful assessment of likely sources of infection can be beneficial to guide appropriate antimicrobial use based on the probable bacteria that reside in those locations. For example, if the source is the gastrointestinal tract, gram-negative bacteria predominate, whereas if the patient has significant skin disease, the antimicrobial therapy should entail drugs with significant gram-positive coverage. In-depth diagnostics beyond a physical examination (such as blood cultures, urine cultures, and advanced imaging) attempting to identify a source of infection often are of little immediate value (because of the length of time needed to culture bacteria and determine susceptibility patterns), and are not routinely performed unless there is a clinical indication for these tests. This inability to instantly identify the inciting infectious organisms and appropriate drug to treat them further justifies the need for a wide spectrum of antimicrobial coverage.

Most patients have infections that are susceptible to standard antimicrobials.[10] However, if a patient is not responding to appropriate antimicrobial therapy within a few doses, reevaluation of the spectrum of activity should be performed and extended to broaden the spectrum of activity (**Table 3**).

SPECIAL CONSIDERATIONS WHEN INITIATING ANTIMICROBIAL THERAPY IN FEBRILE, NEUTROPENIC PATIENTS

Critically ill or septic patients often have special considerations that should be recognized so as to institute appropriate dosing and therapies. In general, pharmacokinetics are critical in drug dosing for high-risk patients.[14] It is extremely important that

Table 3		
Commonly used parenteral antimicrobials		
Gram Positive	Gram Negative	Anaerobes
Ampicillin	Amikacin	Metronidazole
Ampicillin + Sublactam	Gentamicin	
Cefazolin	Enrofloxacin	
Ticarcillin		
Cefoxitin		

Many of the antimicrobials have a broader spectrum of activity than the listed primary category.

antimicrobials are never underdosed, but this is particularly true in critical patients. In fact, altered dosing of certain antimicrobials may be needed to offset the limitations in perfusion that occur in septic patients.[14,15] In human critical patients, some antimicrobials' penetration into tissues can be altered to 5 to 10 times lower than what the penetration would be in a healthy patient.[14,16] Often when managing a febrile neutropenic patient, the author uses the upper end of the recommended dose range in an attempt to ensure the most appropriate antimicrobial concentrations are achieved.

There also are other considerations to assess when selecting an appropriate antimicrobial for a febrile, neutropenic patient. As many antimicrobials are highly protein bound, evaluation of the albumin in patients is of particular importance to help with the most appropriate antimicrobial selection and dose.

Additionally, most chemotherapy patients have been exposed to previous antimicrobials and therefore there is always a concern regarding acquired drug resistance. In fact, increasing resistance to fluoroquinolones is of significant concern and is having a major impact on both the human and veterinary medical profession.[17] Although no studies to date in veterinary medicine have documented a direct link between previous antimicrobial exposure and drug resistance during a febrile, neutropenic episode, the possibility exists and should be carefully considered. This is particularly true if a patient is not responding appropriately or as expected after receiving standard antimicrobial therapy for a febrile neutropenia episode.

In general, most patients with febrile neutropenia will respond to appropriate supportive care within a few hours of initiating care and can be discharged within 24 to 48 hours of initial presentation. Criteria that are often used to determine when it is safe for a patient to be discharged include eating, drinking, afebrile, and acting normally. The neutrophil count should be increasing as well, but the absolute number is not as important as patients are more likely to obtain an infection in a hospital setting as opposed to being in their normal home environment. Patients should be discharged with a course of broad-spectrum antimicrobials to be administered orally at home for at least 3 to 7 additional days.

PROPHYLACTIC ANTIMICROBIAL USE

The prophylactic use of antimicrobials in both human and veterinary oncology is a controversial issue. It has been well-documented in humans that the addition of a fluoroquinolone antimicrobial to drug regimens for patients at high risk of a febrile neutropenia episode is indicated. Prophylactic antimicrobials have been shown to decrease the incidence of fever, infection, and hospitalization of patients.[18] However, more evidence is supporting the notion that patients should be critically evaluated for their risk of a febrile neutropenic episode before dispensing antimicrobials, especially in light of increasing resistance to antimicrobials in human medicine. There is a paucity of information regarding prophylactic use of antimicrobials in veterinary medicine. Prophylactic antimicrobial use in veterinary medicine can be divided into 2 major types: those administered to afebrile, neutropenic patients, and those prescribed to patients after chemotherapy administration to try to prevent an infection.

PROPHYLACTIC ANTIMICROBIAL USE AFTER CHEMOTHERAPY ADMINISTRATION: "PREVENTION ANTIMICROBIALS"

In human oncology, prophylactic prescription of antimicrobials is limited to those patients considered at high risk of developing a febrile neutropenic episode after chemotherapy. In general, this constitutes patients with lymphomas/leukemias, high-dose chemotherapy patients, and first round of treatment for solid tumors or lymphoma.[18,19]

The same considerations could be used for veterinary patients as well. Increased incidence of hospitalization has been documented in dogs after the initial combination treatment of vincristine/L-asparaginase for canine lymphoma.[20] In that study, 16% of patients had to be hospitalized and no factors could be identified as to which patients were at increased risk.[20] Only one prospective study has truly evaluated the prophylactic use and benefit of trimethoprim-sulfadiazine in veterinary patients with osteosarcoma and lymphoma being treated with doxorubicin chemotherapy.[21] This study found a reduction in morbidity associated with prophylactic antimicrobial use in these patients.[21] Other factors have been evaluated to help predict which patients are at an increased risk of potential sepsis (**Box 1**).

However, in general, little other evidence supports the use of prophylactic antimicrobials to prevent an infection in dogs receiving chemotherapy. In fact, a 2012 study documented that of patients that presented for an episode of febrile neutropenia, 22% had been prescribed prophylactic antimicrobials. The use of these antimicrobials did not alter the length of hospital stay or the final outcome of the episode.[13] Often it is a clinical decision based on clinician preference as to whether or not prophylactic antimicrobial usage is warranted to try to prevent an infection in patients receiving chemotherapy.

ANTIMICROBIAL USE IN AFEBRILE, NEUTROPENIC PATIENTS

One of the most common uses of antimicrobials in oncology patients is for those patients that are afebrile, but neutropenic after receiving chemotherapy drugs. The most common nadir for neutrophils after chemotherapy is 5 to 7 days. There are a few drugs that also can have a prolonged or late nadir, including CCNU (lomustine) and carboplatin.[1,3,5–8] In general, patients that feel clinically well, are afebrile, and have more than 1000 neutrophils/μL have little need for antimicrobial coverage. However, if patients are feeling clinically well, afebrile, and have less than 1000 neutrophils/μL, this is traditionally an indication for antimicrobial coverage.[3,4] It is thought that with more than approximately 1000 neutrophils/μL, the risk of an infection is relatively low.[22] Nevertheless, it is important to remember, as previously mentioned, that a complete blood count is a snapshot in time and there is no way to predict if the neutrophil count is going up or down. Therefore, if a patient is borderline on the neutrophil count (<1500 neutrophils/μL) some oncologists will use oral antimicrobials.[3]

In general, antimicrobial selection is largely based on clinician preference and the particular situation.[23] A 2013 study by Regan and colleagues[23] identified commonly used prophylactic antimicrobials by veterinary oncologists in afebrile, neutropenic, but clinically well patients (**Table 4**).[3] For the most part, when using antimicrobials in this scenario, selecting antimicrobials that have a broad spectrum of activity, but

---

Box 1
Factors that may help predict which patients should receive prophylactic antimicrobial use

Small body weight

Induction phase of chemotherapy (particularly lymphoma)

Tumor type (Hematologic)

Chemotherapy drug administered (vincristine or doxorubicin)

Breed (mutation in P-glycoprotein)

Adapted from Refs.[12,20,21]

Table 4
Commonly used antimicrobials for afebrile, neutropenic patients

Antimicrobial	Pros	Cons
Amoxicillin/ clavulanic acid	Broad-spectrum gram-positive, gram-negative, anaerobes Readily available Multiple sizes of tablets available, including liquid Good absorption orally Safe with wide dosing range Bactericidal Most commonly used prophylactic antimicrobial by veterinary oncologists	Cost, particularly for large-breed dogs Anaerobic spectrum of activity Twice daily dosing
Enrofloxacin	Good gram-negative activity, limited activity against other bacteria Readily available Once-a-day dosing Efficacy documented with this class of drug in human oncology Well absorbed orally Bactericidal	Cost Efficacy can decrease with underdosing Potential persistent multidrug resistance developing Cartilage damage in growing dogs Blindness in cats
Trimethoprim sulfa	Broad spectrum of activity: gram positive, gram negative, anaerobes Readily available Efficacy documented with this class of drug in human and veterinary oncology Inexpensive Readily absorbed orally Bactericidal	Side effects: bone marrow suppression, KCS, immune-mediated disease, hypothyroidism Anaerobic activity Twice-daily dosing
Cephalexin	Good gram-positive spectrum of activity Readily available Inexpensive Bactericidal Readily absorbed orally	Limited spectrum of activity Capsule/tablet sizes limited 2–3 times per day dosing

Abbreviation: KCS, keratoconjunctivitis sicca.

spare the anaerobic bacteria is recommended.[4,10,24] In theory, the anaerobic bacteria may assist in the prevention of overgrowth of aerobic bacteria in the gastrointestinal tract.[4,10,24] Because active infection is not present, afebrile, neutropenic patients are commonly placed on 3 to 7 days of antimicrobial coverage.[3,4,10] It is vital to use appropriate doses of antimicrobials to help decrease the development of resistance. Moreover, careful monitoring of the patient over the next few days is of utmost importance. The veterinarian should evaluate any change in attitude, appetite, or gastrointestinal signs immediately, as these could be signs of a patient becoming septic.

ANTIMICROBIAL USE IN RADIATION THERAPY PATIENTS

The uses and indications for radiation therapy in veterinary oncology patients are ever growing. With the increased use, knowledge of common side effects and how to properly manage them is vitally important for these patients. With that in mind, there are several uses for antimicrobials in patients receiving radiation therapy: acute side effects (mucositis, dermatitis, colitis), and concurrent use of chemotherapy and radiation therapy.

Radiation therapy is a local disease treatment that affects only the area being treated. Therefore, side effects are related to local disease. Acute radiation dermatitis is a common side effect experienced with most curative-intent protocols. In general, topical antimicrobials are used by almost 70% of radiation facilities in North America, with the most common being silver sulfadiazine.[25] Topical therapy is frequently initiated at the first sign of radiation-induced dermatitis.[25] In addition to topical therapy for acute radiation dermatitis, oral antimicrobials are sometimes necessary as well. The most common oral antimicrobials are those traditionally used for skin disease, with primarily a gram-positive spectrum of activity, including cephalexin, cefpodoxime, and amoxicillin/clavulanic acid.[25] If head or neck tumors are irradiated, with the oral cavity in the radiation field, patients can also develop inflammation or irritation to the oral cavity known as mucositis. Mucositis is an acute radiation toxicity and is usually treated with supportive care, including antimicrobials. Antimicrobials often chosen are those that would most effectively target the bacteria in the oral cavity, particularly anaerobes. Therefore, amoxicillin/clavulanic acid and clindamycin are 2 of the most commonly used. When the gastrointestinal tract is in the radiation field, patients can develop acute colitis. Colitis is considered another acute radiation side effect that resolves with supportive care after discontinuation of the radiation therapy. Supportive care for colitis often includes metronidazole in combination with other gastrointestinal medications (**Table 5**).

The final indication for antimicrobial usage is when patients are concurrently receiving radiation therapy and chemotherapy. This combination potentially results in a greater risk of myelosuppression, including both neutropenia and thrombocytopenia.[26] A 2009 study by Hume and colleagues[26] evaluating the combination of carboplatin and radiation identified approximately 20% of patients developing significant hematological toxicity. Additionally, 10% of patients developed significant gastrointestinal side effects. Therefore, prophylactic antimicrobials are often clinically used in this situation because of the increased risk of myelosuppression and toxicity.

DOXYCYCLINE AND VETERINARY ONCOLOGY PATIENTS

Doxycycline is a tetracycline antimicrobial that is often used to treat infectious diseases in small animal patients. There are 2 uses of this antimicrobial that impact veterinary oncology patients. Frequently, patients with generalized lymphadenopathy are prescribed doxycycline to treat a potential tick-borne infectious process until a definitive diagnosis can be determined. Early laboratory work conducted by Mealey and colleagues[27] revealed that doxycycline can induce the expression of P-glycoprotein,

Table 5 Antimicrobial use in radiation therapy	
Indications for Antimicrobials in Radiation Therapy Patients	**Antimicrobials Commonly Used**
Acute radiation dermatitis	Topical: silver sulfadiazine, 2% chlorhexidine gluconate solution Oral: cephalexin, cefpodoxime, amoxicillin/clavulanic acid
Acute radiation mucositis	Amoxicillin/clavulanic acid Clindamycin
Acute radiation colitis	Metronidazole
Concurrent chemotherapy and radiation therapy	Amoxicillin/clavulanic acid, enrofloxacin, trimethaprim sulfa, cephalexin

a drug-resistance protein, in human breast cancer cells. The drug-resistance protein, P-glycoprotein, is normally responsible for pumping foreign substances out of cells, particularly steroids and commonly used chemotherapy agents (vinca alkaloids, doxorubicin). Although no in vivo studies have been conducted to date, the potential to increase drug resistance and decrease the efficacy of lymphoma treatments in these patients pretreated with doxycycline theoretically exists.

Doxycycline also has been documented to have some antiangiogenic properties via inhibition of matrix metalloproteinases.[28] Metronomic chemotherapy (ie, low-dose chemotherapy) is thought to indirectly impact angiogenesis through various mechanisms.[29] Therefore, it has been postulated that the addition of doxycycline to some low-dose chemotherapy protocols may be of benefit. However, the addition of minocycline to a standard protocol for dogs with hemangiosarcoma failed to yield a survival benefit compared with those who received chemotherapy alone.[30] This is an area of future study and direction in both human and veterinary oncology. Appropriate dosages and dosing schemes still need further work to determine the ideal treatment plan if doxycycline is to be incorporated into standard low-dose chemotherapy protocols.

REFERENCES

1. Wilson H, Barton C. Chemotherapy. In: Boothe DM, editor. Small animal clinical pharmacology and therapeutics. 2nd edition. St Louis (MO): Elsevier Saunders; 2012. p. 1210–35.
2. Stockham SL, Scott MA. Leukocytes. In: Stockham SL, Scott MA, editors. Fundamentals of veterinary clinical pathology. 2nd edition. Ames (IA): Blackwell Publishing; 2008. p. 53–106.
3. Brugmann B. Neutropenia and sepsis in chemotherapy patients. Stand Care 2008;10(8):3–6.
4. Thamm DH, Vail DM. Aftershocks of cancer chemotherapy: managing adverse effects. J Am Anim Hosp Assoc 2007;43:1–7.
5. Page RL, McEntee MC, George SL, et al. Pharmacokinetic and phase I evaluation of carboplatin in dogs. J Vet Intern Med 1993;7:235–40.
6. Moore AS, London CA, Wood CA, et al. Lomustine (CCNU) for the treatment of resistant lymphoma in dogs. J Vet Intern Med 1999;13:395–8.
7. Saba CF, Vail DM, Thamm DH. Phase II clinical evaluation of lomustine chemotherapy for feline vaccine-associated sarcoma. Vet Comp Oncol 2012;10:283–91.
8. Rassnick KM, Gieger TL, Williams LE, et al. Phase I evaluation of CCNU (lomustine) in tumor-bearing cats. J Vet Intern Med 2001;15:196–9.
9. VCOG. Veterinary Co-operative Oncology Group – common terminology criteria for adverse events (VCOG-CTCAE) following chemotherapy or biological antineoplastic therapy in dogs and cats v1.1. Vet Comp Oncol 2011. http://dx.doi.org/10.1111/j.1476-5829.2011.00283.x.
10. Vail DM. Supporting the veterinary cancer patient on chemotherapy: neutropenia and gastrointestinal toxicity. Top Companion Anim Med 2009;24:122–9.
11. Chun R, Garrett LD, MacEwen EG. In: Withrow SJ, MacEwen EG, editors. Small animal clinical oncology. 3rd edition. St Louis (MO): Elsevier Saunders; 2001. p. 92–118.
12. Sorenmo KU, Harwood LP, King LG, et al. Case-control study to evaluate risk factors for the development of sepsis (neutropenia and fever) in dogs receiving chemotherapy. J Am Vet Med Assoc 2010;236:650–6.
13. Britton BM, Kelleher ME, Gregor TP, et al. Evaluation of factors associated with prolonged hospital stay and outcome of febrile neutropenic patients receiving

chemotherapy: 70 cases (1997-2010). Vet Comp Oncol 2012. http://dx.doi.org/10.1111/vco.12001.

14. Hackett ES, Gustafson DL. Alterations of drug metabolism in critically ill animals. Vet Clin North Am Small Anim Pract 2011;41:805–15.

15. Georges B, Conil JM, Cougot P, et al. Cefepime in critically ill patients: continuous infusion vs. an intermittent dosing regimen. Int J Clin Pharmacol Ther 2005;43:360–9.

16. Joukhadar C, Frossard M, Mayer BX, et al. Impaired target site penetration of beta-lactams may account for therapeutic failure in patients with septic shock. Crit Care Med 2001;29:385–91.

17. Boothe DM. Antimicrobial drugs. In: Boothe DM, editor. Small animal clinical pharmacology and therapeutics. 2nd edition. St Louis (MO): Elsevier Saunders; 2012. p. 189–270.

18. Cullen M, Steven N, Billingham L, et al. Antibacterial prophylaxis after chemotherapy for solid tumors and lymphomas. N Engl J Med 2005;353:988–98.

19. Lo N, Cullen M. Antibiotic prophylaxis in chemotherapy-induced neutropenia: time to reconsider. Hematol Oncol 2006;24:120–5.

20. Northrup NC, Rassnick KM, Snyder LA, et al. Neutropenia associated with vincristine and L-asparaginase induction chemotherapy for canine lymphoma. J Vet Intern Med 2002;16:570–5.

21. Chretin JD, Rassnick KM, Shaw NA, et al. Prophylactic trimethoprim-sulfadiazine during chemotherapy in dogs with lymphoma and osteosarcoma: a double-blind, placebo-controlled study. J Vet Intern Med 2007;21:141–8.

22. Couto CG. Management of complications of chemotherapy. Vet Clin North Am Small Anim Pract 1990;20:1037–53.

23. Regan RC, Kaplan MS, Bailey DB. Diagnostic evaluation and treatment recommendations for dogs with substage-a high-grade multicentric lymphoma: results of a survey of veterinarians. Vet Comp Oncol 2013;11:287–95.

24. Waaij D. The colonization resistance of the digestive tract in experimental animals and its consequences for infection prevention, acquisition of new bacteria and the prevention of spread of bacteria between cage mates. In: Waaij D, Verhoef J, editors. New criteria for antimicrobial therapy: maintenance of digestive tract colonization resistance. Excerpta Medica International Congress Series. Amsterdam: Elsevier; 1979. p. 43–53.

25. Flynn DK, Lurie DM. Canine acute radiation dermatitis, a survey of current management practices in North America. Vet Comp Oncol 2007;5:197–207.

26. Hume KR, Johnson JL, Williams LE. Adverse effects of concurrent carboplatin chemotherapy and radiation therapy in dogs. J Vet Intern Med 2009;23:24–30.

27. Mealey KL, Barhoumi R, Burghardt RC, et al. Doxycycline induces expression of P glycoprotein in MCF-7 breast carcinoma cells. Antimicrobial Agents Chemother 2002;46:755–61.

28. Sapadin AN, Fleischmajer R. Tetracyclines: nonantibiotic properties and their clinical implications. J Am Acad Dermatol 2006;54:258–65.

29. Mutsaers AJ. Metronomic chemotherapy. Top Companion Anim Med 2009;24:137–43.

30. Sorenmo K, Duda L, Barber L, et al. Canine hemangiosarcoma treated with standard chemotherapy and minocycline. J Vet Intern Med 2000;14:395–8.

Small Molecule Inhibitors in Veterinary Oncology Practice

Cheryl A. London, DVM, PhD

KEYWORDS

- Dog • Protein • Kinase • Inhibitor

KEY POINTS

- Recent advances in molecular biology have permitted the identification and characterization of specific abnormalities regarding cell signaling and function in cancer cells.
- Proteins that are found to be dysregulated in cancer cells can serve as relevant targets for therapeutic intervention.
- Although there are several approaches to block proteins that contribute to cellular dysfunction, the one most commonly used involves a class of therapeutics called small molecule inhibitors.
- Such inhibitors work by disrupting critical pathways/processes in cancer cells, thereby disrupting their ability to grow and survive.
- There are now 2 small molecule inhibitors approved/conditionally approved for use in veterinary medicine, toceranib (Palladia) and masitinib (Kinavet), and it is likely several more will be approved in the future.

INTRODUCTION

With recent advances in genetics and molecular techniques, key proteins that contribute to dysregulation of cancer cells are now being identified and characterized. These proteins play essential roles in regulating cell survival, growth, differentiation, and migration, among other processes. Although many of the proteins found to be abnormal in cancer cells are kinases that phosphorylate other proteins in the cell and are integral components of cell signaling, others are transcription factors, proteins that block apoptosis (cell death), heat shock proteins, and regulators of nuclear export, among others. Given their known role in driving the development and progression of tumors, substantial effort has been directed at blocking the function of these proteins. Monoclonal antibodies are primarily directed at cell surface proteins, and

Veterinary Biosciences, The Ohio State University, 454 VMAB, 1925 Coffey Road, Columbus, OH 43210, USA
E-mail address: london.20@osu.edu

Vet Clin Small Anim 44 (2014) 893–908
http://dx.doi.org/10.1016/j.cvsm.2014.06.001
0195-5616/14/$ – see front matter © 2014 Elsevier Inc. All rights reserved.

small molecule inhibitors are capable of targeting proteins on the cell surface, in the cytoplasm, and in the nucleus.

A variety of small molecule inhibitors have been approved for the treatment of human cancers. In some instances, these inhibitors have exhibited significant clinical efficacy and it is likely their biological activity will be further enhanced as combination regimens with standard treatment modalities are explored. In veterinary medicine, the use of small molecule inhibitors is relatively recent, although 2 inhibitors, toceranib (Palladia; Zoetis, Madison, NJ, USA) and masitinib (Kinavet; Catalent Pharma Solutions, Somerset, NJ, USA), have been approved or conditionally approved by the US Food and Drug Administration (FDA) for use in dogs.[1,2]

REGULATION OF NORMAL CELL BIOLOGY

The signals and processes that regulate normal cell biology, including survival, growth, and differentiation, are tightly regulated. Cells receive a multitude of signals from their environment that are processed continuously, and the sum of these signals ultimately shapes cell fate. Signals received by cells include those generated by growth factors (GFs), cytokines, electrolytes, cell-cell contact, and the extracellular matrix, among others.

One of the best-described types of signaling involves a class of proteins called kinases. These kinases act through phosphorylation of other proteins by binding adenosine triphosphate (ATP) and adding phosphate groups to key amino acids on themselves (also known as autophosphorylation) and on other proteins, thereby promoting the transmission of cellular signals.[3] This process usually occurs following stimuli generated by GFs or other substances outside of the cell. They are termed tyrosine kinases (TKs) if they phosphorylate proteins on tyrosine or serine/threonine kinases if they phosphorylate proteins on serine and threonine. Receptor tyrosine kinases (RTKs) are TKs expressed on the cell surface stimulated by binding of GFs (**Fig. 1**). Signaling generated by kinases is a major driver of normal cell differentiation, survival, and growth. RTKs, including vascular endothelial growth factor receptor (VEGFR), platelet-derived growth factor receptor (PDGFR), fibroblast growth factor receptor

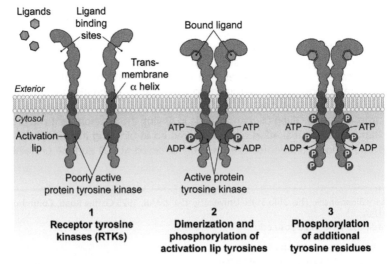

Fig. 1. RTKs are expressed on the cell surface and are stimulated by binding of GFs.

(FGFR), and Tie-1 and Tie-2 (receptors for angiopoietin), are also important in the process of angiogenesis, which is critical for tumors to grow beyond a few millimeters in size.[4–7]

Two cytoplasmic pathways known to be key players in normal cell signaling are the RAF/MAPK (RAS-RAF-MEK-ERK/p38/JNK family members, **Fig. 2**),[8,9] and the phosphatidyl inositol-3 kinase pathway (PI3K, AKT, NFkB, and mTOR, among others, see **Fig. 2**).[10,11] These pathways have previously been reviewed in detail. Specific members of the RAS/MAPK pathway known to be mutated in human tumors include RAS (lung cancer, colon cancer, and several hematologic malignancies) and BRAF (melanomas and thyroid carcinomas, colon cancer).[8,12,13] Abnormalities of PI3K including mutations and gene amplification are found in many human cancers, including breast, colorectal, lung, and ovarian carcinomas.[14] Loss of activity of PTEN, a phosphatase that normally acts to regulate AKT and terminate signaling,[11,15,16] can also activate this pathway. PTEN mutations and/or decreased PTEN expression occur in many human cancers (eg, glioblastoma and prostate cancer)[14,15] and have been documented in canine cancers as well (osteosarcoma [OSA], melanoma).[17–19]

Ultimately, signal transduction influences cellular events by altering the functions of key transcription factors that either induce or repress gene expression, by changing the status of proteins critical to regulation of cell cycling, and through the modulation of the genome itself via epigenetic changes. These processes must be coordinated so as to maintain cellular homeostasis, as well as normal functioning of the organism as a whole.

Dysregulation of Proteins in Cancer Cells

Dysfunction of proteins occurs frequently in cancers, typically through mutation, overexpression, the generation of fusion proteins, and/or the presence of autocrine loops of activation. Mutations often alter the structure of a protein, inducing activation in the absence of an appropriate stimulus. In many cases, the protein dysrgulated is a kinase, resulting in constitutive (unregulated) intracellular signaling. Other classes of proteins that are frequently altered in tumor cells include transcription factors,

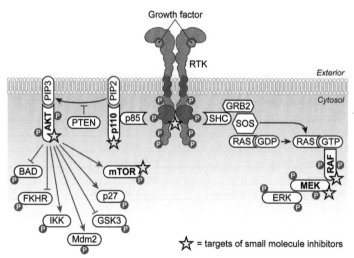

Fig. 2. Two cytoplasmic pathways known to be key players in normal cell signaling are the RAS/RAF/MAPK and PI3K/AKT pathways.

regulators of chromatin structure, and inhibitors of apoptosis. Examples of proteins known to be altered in human and canine cancers are found in **Table 1**.

Small Molecule Kinase Inhibitors: The Human Experience

With the understanding that certain molecular events can act as drivers of uncontrolled cancer cell growth and survival, substantial effort has been directed at blocking the specific proteins that initiate this process either directly at the level of the tumor cell or indirectly at the level of the tumor microenvironment. Although monoclonal antibodies have been developed that target proteins expressed on the cell surface or in the serum/plasma, small molecule inhibitors are designed to target proteins on the cell surface, in the cytoplasm, and in the nucleus. Unlike monoclonal antibodies that are given by injection, most small molecule inhibitors are orally bioavailable and administered on a continual basis. Small molecule inhibitors typically work by blocking the ATP binding site of key proteins (particularly kinases), essentially acting as competitive inhibitors and disrupting their ability to function. They may also block protein-protein interactions, known as allosteric inhibition. **Table 2** provides a list of several small molecule inhibitors that have been approved by the FDA to treat human cancers.

Table 1 Mutations identified in various tumor types	
Tumor Type	**Mutations Identified**
Human cutaneous melanoma	Point mutation BRAF (60% of human tumors) KIT mutations
Hematopoietic neoplasms, lung cancer, colon cancer, others	Point mutation RAS
Canine mast cell tumor (30% high grade)	Internal tandem duplications juxtamembrane domain KIT (exon 11) or extracellular ligand binding domain (exon 8)
GIST (50%–80% human tumors, some dog tumors)	Deletions juxtamembrane domain KIT
AML, acute myelogenous leukemia	FLT-3 internal tandem duplications
Lung carcinomas	EGFR point mutations
Various carcinomas	PI3Ka
Breast & ovarian carcinomas	HER2/neu overexpression
Lung, bladder, cervical, ovarian, renal, pancreatic	EGFR (up to 60 gene copies/cell)
CML (90% of patients)	BCR-ABL fusion protein
Leukemia	TEL-PDGFRβ
Non-small cell lung cancer	EML4-ALK
Burkitt lymphoma	Myc-Igh
Glioblastoma & squamous cell carcinoma	TGFβ and EGFR
Breast & colorectal cancer	IGF (insulinlike growth factor) and IGF1R
Melanoma & glioblastoma	VEGF and VEGFR
Canine OSA	MET and HGF
Canine hemangiosarcoma	KIT and SCF

Data from Refs.[8,15,20–54]

Table 2
Small molecule inhibitors currently approved by the FDA

Agent	Targets	FDA-Approved Indications
Axitinib (Inlyta)	KIT, PDGFRβ, VEGFR1/2/3	Renal cell carcinoma
Bortezomib (Velcade)	Proteasome	Multiple myeloma Mantle cell lymphoma
Bosutinib (Bosulif)	ABL	CML (Philadelphia chromosome positive, Ph+)
Cabozantinib (Cometriq)	FLT3, KIT, MET, RET, VEGFR2	Medullary thyroid cancer
Crizotinib (Xalkori)	ALK, MET	Non-small cell lung cancer (ALK fusion)
Dasatinib (Sprycel)	ABL	CML (Ph+) Acute lymphoblastic leukemia (ALL, Ph+)
Erlotinib (Tarceva)	EGFR (HER1/ERBB1)	Non-small cell lung cancer Pancreatic cancer
Everolimus (Afinitor)	mTOR	Pancreatic neuroendocrine tumor Renal cell carcinoma Subependymal giant cell astrocytoma associated with tuberous sclerosis
Gefitinib (Iressa)	EGFR (HER1/ERBB1)	Non-small cell lung cancer
Imatinib (Gleevec)	KIT, PDGFR, ABL	GIST Dermatofibrosarcoma protuberans Multiple hematologic malignancies including Ph+ ALL and CML
Lapatinib (Tykerb)	HER2 (ERBB2/neu), EGFR (HER1/ERBB1)	Breast cancer (HER2+)
Nilotinib (Tasigna)	ABL	CML (Ph+)
Pazopanib (Votrient)	VEGFR, PDGFR, KIT	Renal cell carcinoma
Ponatinib (Iclusig)	ABL, FGFR1–3, FLT3, VEGFR2	CML and AML (Ph+)
Regorafenib (Stivarga)	KIT, PDGFRβ, RAF, RET, VEGFR1/2/3	Colorectal cancer GIST
Romidepsin (Istodax)	HDAC	Cutaneous T-cell lymphoma
Ruxolitinib (Jakafi)	JAK1/2	Myelofibrosis
Sorafenib (Nexavar)	VEGFR, PDGFR, KIT, RAF	Hepatocellular carcinoma Renal cell carcinoma
Sunitinib (Sutent)	VEGFR, PDGFR, KIT, RET	GIST Dermatofibrosarcoma protuberans Hematologic malignancies including Ph+ ALL and CML Pancreatic neuroendocrine tumor Renal cell carcinoma
Temsirolimus (Torisel)	mTOR	Renal cell carcinoma
Vandetanib (Caprelsa)	EGFR (HER1/ERBB1), RET, VEGFR2	Medullary thyroid cancer
Vemurafenib (Zelboraf)	BRAF	Melanoma (BRAF V600 mutation)
Vorinostat (Zolinza)	HDAC	Cutaneous T-cell lymphoma

SMALL MOLECULE INHIBITORS IN VETERINARY MEDICINE
Toceranib (Palladia)

Toceranib phosphate is an orally bioavailable small molecule inhibitor that blocks a variety of RTKs expressed on the cell surface by acting as a reversible competitive inhibitor of ATP binding, thereby preventing receptor phosphorylation and subsequent downstream signaling. Toceranib's published inhibitory profile includes the RTKs VEGFR2, PDGFRβ, and KIT.[2,20–22] However, it is very closely related to sunitinib (Sutent) that blocks the activity of VEGFR2, VEGFR3, PDGFRα/β, KIT, CSF1R, FLT-3, and RET.[23] A kinome analysis was performed that evaluates the activity of a drug against the more than 500 known human kinases to determine whether the drug can block phosphorylation of these targets (London and colleagues, unpublished data, 2010). These results support the broad activity of toceranib against the split kinase RTKs, RET, and possibly JAK family members. Toceranib was initially developed as an anti-angiogenic agent, as inhibition of VEGFR and PDGFR family members blocks angiogenesis in several mouse tumor models. However, its broad target profile including KIT and FLT-3 results in direct antitumor activity as well. The combination of anti-angiogenic and antitumor activity likely provides more extensive clinical activity than that observed with narrowly targeted small molecule inhibitors.

Toceranib in the Clinic

Phase 1 clinical trial

The first evaluation of toceranib in veterinary medicine was a phase I clinical trial in 57 dogs with a variety of cancers.[20] In this study, objective responses occurred in 16 dogs: 6 complete responses (CR) and 10 partial responses (PR) with stable disease (SD) in an additional 15 dogs for an overall biological activity of 54%. Tumor types that responded to therapy included sarcomas, carcinomas, melanomas, myeloma, and mast cell tumor (MCT)s. As predicted based on the known involvement of KIT dysregulation in canine MCTs, the highest response rate occurred in this disease, with 10 of 11 dogs with KIT mutations exhibiting clinical benefit. The maximum tolerated dose (MTD) was established as 3.25 mg/kg every other day (EOD).

Results of the field study

Based on the phase I study findings, a placebo-controlled randomized clinical field study was subsequently performed in dogs with nonresectable grade 2 and 3 MCTs.[2] During the blinded phase, the response rate in toceranib-treated (n = 86) dogs was 37.2% (7 CR, 25 PR) versus 7.9% (5 PR) in placebo-treated (n = 63) dogs. Of 58 dogs that received toceranib following placebo-escape, 41.4% (8 CR, 16 PR) experienced an objective response. The response rate for all 145 dogs was 42.8% (21 CR, 41 PR) with an additional 16 dogs experiencing SD for an overall biological activity of 60%. Dogs whose MCT had mutations in KIT were twice as likely to respond as those without (69% vs 37%) and dogs without lymph node metastasis had a higher response rate than those with involvement (67% vs 46%).

Biological activity off label

After FDA approval, toceranib was used off label to treat several types of canine cancers, often after failure of primary or standard of care treatments. In retrospective analysis of this use biological activity was observed in several solid tumors including anal gland anal sac adenocarcinoma (AGASACA), metastatic OSA, thyroid carcinoma (thyroid CA), head and neck carcinoma, and nasal carcinoma.[24] Clinical benefit (CR, PR, or SD) was found in 63 of 85 (74%) dogs, including 28 of 32 AGASACA (8 PR, 20 SD), 11 of 23 OSA (1 PR, 10 SD), 12 of 15 thyroid CA (4 PR, 8 SD), 7 of 8 head and neck carcinomas (1 CR, 5 PR, 1 SD), and 5 of 7 (1 CR, 4 SD) nasal carcinomas. For dogs experiencing clinical benefit, the median dose of toceranib used was 2.8 mg/kg; 36/63 (58.7%) patients were given the drug 3 times per week (Monday/Wednesday/Friday) instead of EOD, and 47 of 63 (74.6%) received toceranib for 4 months or longer. Recently, a dog with lymphangiosarcoma that had failed both doxorubicin treatment and metronomic therapy with chlorambucil and meloxicam underwent near complete regression of disease after toceranib therapy.[25] In another case report, a dog with chronic monocytic leukemia exhibited a partial response to toceranib and prednisone.[26] These data, combined with that in the phase 1 study, support the notion that toceranib has biological activity against certain solid tumors (particularly carcinomas) and perhaps some types of leukemia. Clinical trials are underway to help more accurately define this activity.

Combination therapy with piroxicam
Piroxicam, a mixed COX-1/COX-2 inhibitor, has shown some activity in certain carcinomas (transitional cell carcinoma, squamous cell carcinoma) and is often used as part of a metronomic chemotherapy regimen in combination with cyclophosphamide. A phase I trial in tumor-bearing (non-MCT) dogs established the safety of toceranib/piroxicam coadministration[27] at standard dosages (toceranib 3.25 mg/kg EOD and piroxicam 0.3 mg/kg/d) without noting an increase in the frequency of dose-limiting side effects that required discontinuation of therapy. In addition, several antitumor responses were observed. However, the dogs were not monitored to assess whether gastrointestinal (GI) side effects occurred after several months of administration. Therefore, piroxicam is often administered EOD, alternating with toceranib to help mitigate toxicity risk.

Combination therapy with vinblastine
To assess whether vinblastine and toceranib could be effectively combined in the clinical setting, a phase I clinical trial was performed in dogs with MCT.[28] The dose-limiting toxicity for the toceranib/vinblastine combination was neutropenia, and the MTD of vinblastine was 1.6 mg/m^2 every other week when administered with toceranib at 3.25 mg/kg EOD. The 50% reduction in dose intensity for vinblastine was required because of enhancement of myelosuppression when combined with toceranib. Despite the reduction in vinblastine, the objective response rate was 71%, suggesting an additive or possibly synergistic activity with this combination.

Combination therapy with radiation
Radiation therapy is often used following incomplete surgical excision of MCT, but is not considered to be very effective as the sole treatment of gross MCT disease. A clinical trial was performed in which dogs with nonresectable MCTs received prednisone, omeprazole, diphenhydramine, and toceranib at 2.75 mg/kg on Monday/Wednesday/Friday for 1 week before starting coarse-fractionated (6 Gy once per week for 4 weeks) radiation therapy.[29] The objective response rate was 76.4%, with 58.8% of dogs achieving CR and 17.6% achieving PR. The overall median survival time was not reached with a median follow-up of 374 days, suggesting this regimen may have significant clinical benefit in unresectable MCT. Importantly, there was no evidence of enhanced radiation-induced toxicities.

Role in metronomic therapy
Historically, metronomic treatment regimens have included low doses of cyclophosphamide given on a daily basis, often in combination with piroxicam. In dogs with cancer, metronomic cyclophosphamide modulates the number and activity of regulatory

T cells (Tregs) thought to contribute to immune suppression and may therefore be useful in helping to generate an antitumor immune response.[30] Sunitinib, the close counterpart to toceranib, modulates the immune system by reducing the number and function of another immunosuppressive class of cells called myeloid derived suppressor cells,[31] suggesting that at least some of the action of sunitinib may be via enhanced antitumor immunity. Dogs with cancer that received toceranib at 2.75 mg/kg EOD for 2 weeks[32] had significantly reduced numbers and percentages of Treg in the peripheral blood, with a concomitant increase in interferon-γ serum concentrations. Interestingly, the addition of low-dose cyclophosphamide after 2 weeks did not augment this effect. These data indicate that toceranib may be a useful adjunct in metronomic therapy.

Toceranib Dosing

The label dose of toceranib is 3.25 mg/kg EOD based on the clinical field study, with dose reductions in the setting of adverse events. However, evidence exists that good biological activity occurs when doses are initiated less than 3.25 mg/kg. For example, in the phase I study of 16 dogs treated with toceranib at 2.5 mg/kg EOD, 6 of 16 (37.5%) responded to therapy (4 CR, 2 PR), while an additional 5 dogs had SD.[20] This result compared favorably with 20 dogs treated with 3.25 mg/kg EOD in which 8 dogs (40%) had objective responses (2 CR and 6 PR) and an additional 4 dogs had SD. Therefore, the overall biological activity in the 2.5 mg/kg group was 68% compared with 60% in the 3.25 mg/kg group.

These findings are now supported by a prospective study in dogs with solid tumors that found doses of toceranib ranging from 2.4 to 2.9 mg/kg EOD were associated with drug exposure considered sufficient for target inhibition (peak plasma levels of 100–200 ng/mL).[33] Importantly, this lower dosing regimen was associated with a substantially reduced adverse event profile compared with the label dose, with no grade 3 or 4 GI toxicity noted. Moreover, good clinical activity was observed, with both PR and CRs observed, and 35 of 40 dogs remained on toceranib for an average duration of 4 months.[33] With respect to the dosing regimen, toceranib approval was based on EOD administration. Data generated from the retrospective analysis of toceranib use in solid tumors found that 3 times per week dosing may be better tolerated by some dogs and may be particularly useful when toceranib is combined with other therapeutics, such as sonsteroidal anti-inflammatory drugs. Although anecdotal data support this regimen, future studies are needed to confirm that it is comparable to EOD dosing.

Masitinib (Kinavet) and Imatinib

The second small molecule inhibitor conditionally approved for use in dogs is masitinib mesylate (Kinavet), which blocks the activity of KIT, PDGFR, and the cytoplasmic kinase Lyn. A placebo-controlled clinical trial was performed in more than 200 dogs with MCTs in which masitinib significantly improved time to progression, and outcome was improved in dogs with MCTs possessing KIT mutations.[1] Subsequent follow-up of patients treated with masitinib for 1 to 2 years identified an increased number of patients with long-term disease control compared with those treated with placebo (40% vs 15% alive at 2 years).[34] More recently, a retrospective analysis of dogs with MCT treated with masitinib[35] revealed an overall response rate of approximately 50%. Although the number of dogs evaluated in this study was small and they had varying disease presentations, the data indicate that the biological activity of masitinib is likely higher in the setting of primary rather than relapsed disease, and that dogs responding to masitinib may experience long progression-free survivals. Masitinib has also been anecdotally reported to have activity against T-cell lymphoma in dogs.

There have been no formal clinical trials of imatinib mesylate (Gleevec) in veterinary medicine, although a few small studies have been published. In 3 reports, imatinib was well tolerated, and objective antitumor responses were observed in dogs with both mutant and wild-type KIT.[36–38] Responses have also been observed in cats with MCT that have KIT mutations.[39,40] Last, a dog with nonresectable gastrointestinal stromal tumor (GIST) harboring a KIT mutation responded to imatinib therapy.[41]

Management of Adverse Events Associated with Toceranib and Masitinib

Nearly all small molecule inhibitors that have been tested in human patients with cancer induce some adverse events. For many of these drugs, fatigue, lethargy, loss of appetite, and GI effects such as diarrhea are common. Some inhibitors have specific toxicities, including hand-foot syndrome with sunitinib and the development of secondary cutaneous squamous cell carcinoma with vemurafenib, among others. The clinical effects of toceranib and masitinib have been primarily studied in dogs and in most cases they are concordant with those observed in people. It is also important to note that dogs with cancer may have underlying comorbidities that predispose them to some of the toxicities induced by small molecule inhibitors, and as such efforts should be made to improve the health status of dogs before initiation of treatment. This predisposition to some of the toxicities is particularly true for MCT patients who may have subclinical (or clinical) GI ulceration, making them more susceptible to vomiting, diarrhea, and GI bleeding.

For both toceranib and masitinib, the most common adverse events relate to the GI tract, including loss of appetite, diarrhea, and occasionally vomiting.[1,2,20,33,35] The administration of an antacid, particularly omeprazole, may be beneficial in mitigating the risk of GI ulceration, particularly in the setting of MCT. Inappetence is a relatively common side effect and typically responds to standard antinausea therapies (metoclopramide, ondansetron, maropitant) or the addition of low-dose (0.5 mg/kg) prednisone. With respect to diarrhea, metronidazole and/or loperamide are often useful, particularly if the diarrhea is intermittent. In some cases, dogs may require continual administration of metronidazole to prevent break-through episodes while on treatment.

Other toxicities have been observed with the use of toceranib and masitinib in dogs, although these tend to occur with a much lower frequency than those associated with the GI tract. Hepatotoxicity has been reported with a variety of small molecule inhibitors used in people and has also been identified in dogs receiving both toceranib and masitinib. The mechanism for this side effect is not entirely clear, although in the author's experience, it responds to the addition of denamarin and a drug holiday; occasionally, a dose or regimen change is also instituted. Neutropenia has also been noted with both drugs, although it is rarely clinically relevant and typically does not require discontinuation of therapy. Other rare effects include muscle pain and coagulopathies.

Both protein losing nephropathy (PLN) and hypertension have been associated with toceranib administration. In human patients with cancer that receive sunitinib, the incidence of PLN has been reported to be approximately 2.5%.[42–44] The mechanisms through which vascular endothelial growth factor (VEGF)/VEGFR signaling inhibitors cause proteinuria are not well understood, but several have been proposed including the loss of healthy, fenestrated glomerular capillaries, which seems to be a direct consequence of blocking VEGFR signaling and possibly disruption of podocyte integrity.[42–44] In the author's experience, the PLN is generally mild to moderate and typically effectively managed with enalapril/benazepril and/or dose reduction. Similarly, the hypertension can be treated with antihypertensives such as amlodipine.

Masitinib has also been reported to induce PLN, although a much more serious and sometimes fatal condition of protein loss can occur in rare cases, sometimes resulting in death.[35,45] The mechanism of this syndrome is not apparent, although damage to both podocytes and renal tubules was noted in one dog that underwent necropsy. Last, although pancreatitis has been reported following toceranib therapy, this side effect is not clearly linked to drug administration and was not identified in dogs treated with the lower dosing regimen. Should it occur during treatment, once resolved, reinstitution of the drug should be undertaken with caution. For both toceranib and masitinib, drug holiday, dose reduction, and schedule modification represent extremely useful tools in managing clinical toxicities and should be instituted as needed in conjunction with the use of concomitant medications.

Additional Small Molecule Inhibitors Under Investigation

Although kinases have represented the major target for therapeutic intervention with small molecule inhibitors, several other proteins are critical players in cancer cell growth and survival. Small molecules that target these proteins have been evaluated in human clinical trials, and some are now approved for use, including bortezamib (Velcade, targeting the proteasome; Millenium Pharmaceuticals, Cambridge, MA, USA) and vorinostat (Zolinza, a histone deacetylase [HDAC] inhibitor; Merck, Whitehouse Station, NJ, USA), among others. More recently, some of these novel small molecule inhibitors have been tested in dogs with cancer.

STA-1474 is a highly soluble prodrug of ganetespib (formerly STA-9090), a novel resorcinol-containing compound unrelated to geldanamycin that binds in the ATP-binding domain at the N-terminus of HSP90 and acts as a potent HSP90 inhibitor.[46] This prodrug prevents the stabilization of several client proteins (including KIT, MET, BRAF, AKT, among others), ultimately resulting in their degradation. A phase I clinical trial of STA-1474 was performed in dogs with cancer.[47] In this study, 25 dogs were enrolled and objective responses occurred in dogs with MCT (n = 3), OSA (n = 1), oral malignant melanoma (n = 1), and metastatic thyroid carcinoma (n = 1), for a response rate of 24% (6/25). Stable disease (>10 weeks) was seen in 3 dogs, for a resultant overall biological activity of 36% (9/25). Toxicities were nearly all grade 1 and grade 2 and consisted primarily of diarrhea, vomiting, inappetence, and lethargy that were effectively managed with concomitant medications. A subsequent regimen-finding clinical trial was conducted in dogs with MCT, demonstrating that 2-day-in-a-row dosing was most effective with all dogs in this cohort exhibiting reduction in tumor size.

Exportin 1 (XPO1) is a member of the karyopherin family of transport receptors that binds approximately 220 target proteins through a nuclear export signal present in the cargo, resulting in nuclear export.[48] XPO1 is the sole nuclear exporter of several major tumor suppressor and growth regulatory proteins[49,50] and its expression is up-regulated in both hematologic malignancies and solid tumors, often correlating with a poor prognosis,[51–53] KPT-335 (verdinexor) is a novel selective inhibitor of nuclear export (SINE) compound that is an orally bioavailable small molecule inhibitor of XPO1. SINE compounds similar to KPT-335 induce apoptosis and block proliferation in several cancer cell lines,[49,54–56] while sparing normal cells.[57] Additional studies have shown potent anticancer activity and good tolerability of SINE compounds in mouse human xenograft models. A phase I study of KPT-335 was undertaken in dogs with cancer, with enrichment for dogs with non-Hodgkin lymphoma (NHL) based on in vitro studies.[58] The MTD was 1.75 mg/kg given orally twice per week (Monday/Thursday), although biological activity was observed at 1 mg/kg. Clinical benefit, including PR to therapy (n = 2) and SD (n = 7), was observed in 9 of 14 dogs with NHL. A dose expansion study was performed in 6 dogs with NHL given 1.5 mg/kg KPT-335 Monday/Wednesday/Friday;

clinical benefit was observed in 4 of 6 dogs. Toxicities were primarily GI, consisting of anorexia, weight loss, vomiting, and diarrhea and were manageable with supportive care, dose modulation, and administration of low-dose prednisone. Verdinexor is currently undergoing clinical development for the treatment of canine NHL. Importantly, these studies laid the groundwork for the current phase 1 evaluation of the SINE compound KPT-330 (selinexor) in humans with cancer.

HDAC enzymes are responsible for the removal of acetyl groups from the NH_2-terminal tails of histone proteins and play a crucial role in the control of gene expression.[59] Significant interest exists in the use of HDAC inhibitors (HDACi) to treat cancer because this therapy can alter the expression of epigenetically silenced genes in tumor cells and thereby inhibit tumor progression.[60,61] Many HDACi have shown antitumor activity either alone or in chemotherapy combinations. The antiepileptic drug valproic acid, belonging to the short-chain fatty acid class of HDACi, has also demonstrated activity in several tumor models, particularly in combination therapy.[62–64] Previous work demonstrated that the pretreatment of canine and human OSA cells with valproic acid sensitized them to doxorubicin, resulting in decreased proliferation and increased apoptosis; this was confirmed in a xenograft model of canine OSA.[65] Based on these results, a phase 1 study of oral valproic acid was conducted in dogs with cancer when given in combination with a standard dose of doxorubicin.[66] A sustained-release formulation of valproic acid was administered 48 hours before doxorubicin. Trough valproic acid level increased linearly with the dose administered. In addition, there was no evidence that the use of valproic acid altered AUC, half-life, or clearance of doxorubicin. Valproic acid also did not result in significant myelosuppression nor did it potentiate doxorubicin-induced myelosuppression at valproic acid doses up to 240 mg/kg/d. Target modulation as evidenced by histone H3 hyperacetylation was demonstrated in both normal and tumor tissues and the magnitude of hyperacetylation correlated positively with the administered dose of valproic acid. Objective responses were observed in this study, and a few responses were seen in traditionally anthracycline-resistant tumors. The combination was safe and well tolerated, setting the stage for future clinical work with this drug combination.

Resistance to Small Molecule Inhibitors

In people, the response of tumor cells to small molecule inhibitors in the presence of known protein dysregulation is often dramatic, with objective response rates often exceeding 50%, far higher than typically observed with chemotherapy alone. Unfortunately, in most cases, these responses are not durable, lasting from 6 to 18 months on average before relapse. The mechanisms that drive resistance to small molecule inhibitors have been well characterized for specific therapeutics, such as imatinib and erlotinib, but remain only partly understood for many others.[67] In general, more than one cellular alteration contributes to drug resistance, complicating strategies to prevent or circumvent this issue.

Perhaps the most intensively investigated mechanism of drug resistance is that associated with imatinib treatment of BCR-ABL-positive chronic myelogenous leukemia (CML).[68,69] For patients that take imatinib, the primary cause for relapse is the development of point mutations in the protein that often prevents imatinib binding. In addition, some patients develop resistance through up-regulation of BCR-ABL mRNA, resulting in protein overexpression that overwhelms the ability of imatinib to block function.[70] Last, elevated p-glycoprotein expression and enhanced multidrug efflux, as well as activation of other growth factor pathways, have been documented in some patients.

For patients with mutations in epidermal growth factor receptor (EGFR) that respond to the EGFR inhibitor erlotinib, resistance to therapy is mediated by 3 different mechanisms.[71] The first is the generation of a second mutation in the EGFR ATP-binding pocket (T790M) that hinders drug binding. The second involves amplification of the gene encoding MET, which up-regulates MET protein expression, causing phosphorylation through heterodimerization with ERBB3 (another EGFR family member) that sustains signaling downstream, thus circumventing the erlotinib's inhibition of EGFR signaling. Last, overexpression of HGF, the ligand for MET, has been documented in some patients that received erlotinib, resulting in MET phosphorylation and signaling that is independent of EGFR.

Other mechanisms of resistance to kinase inhibitors that are not as well characterized include epigenetic changes secondary to alterations in histone acetylation/deacetylation and chromatin and histone methylation.[67] These changes act to modify the expression of genes that regulate responsiveness to kinase inhibitors, thus promoting escape from therapy.

SUMMARY

Progress in molecular biology has permitted a greater understanding of how protein dysregulation in tumor cells drives uncontrolled growth and survival. The development of small molecule inhibitors that target these key proteins has transformed human cancer therapy. The use of such agents is just beginning to be explored in veterinary oncology and this process has been accelerated through the approval of both toceranib and masitinib. Nevertheless, significant challenges remain, including determining how these therapies can be effectively combined with chemotherapy and radiation therapy to provide optimal anticancer efficacy without enhancing toxicity, and identifying strategies that are less likely to result in drug resistance.

REFERENCES

1. Hahn KA, Ogilvie G, Rusk T, et al. Masitinib is safe and effective for the treatment of canine mast cell tumors. J Vet Intern Med 2008;22:1301–9.
2. London CA, Malpas PB, Wood-Follis SL, et al. Multi-center, placebo-controlled, double-blind, randomized study of oral toceranib phosphate (SU11654), a receptor tyrosine kinase inhibitor, for the treatment of dogs with recurrent (either local or distant) mast cell tumor following surgical excision. Clin Cancer Res 2009;15:3856–65.
3. Lemmon MA, Schlessinger J. Cell signaling by receptor tyrosine kinases. Cell 2010;141:1117–34.
4. Cherrington JM, Strawn LM, Shawver LK. New paradigms for the treatment of cancer: the role of anti- angiogenesis agents. Adv Cancer Res 2000;79:1–38.
5. Eskens FA. Angiogenesis inhibitors in clinical development; where are we now and where are we going? Br J Cancer 2004;90:1–7.
6. McCarty MF, Liu W, Fan F, et al. Promises and pitfalls of anti-angiogenic therapy in clinical trials. Trends Mol Med 2003;9:53–8.
7. Thurston G. Role of angiopoietins and tie receptor tyrosine kinases in angiogenesis and lymphangiogenesis. Cell Tissue Res 2003;314:61–8.
8. Downward J. Targeting RAS signalling pathways in cancer therapy. Nat Rev Cancer 2003;3:11–22.
9. Johnson GL, Lapadat R. Mitogen-activated protein kinase pathways mediated by ERK, JNK, and p38 protein kinases. Science 2002;298:1911–2.
10. Franke TF, Hornik CP, Segev L, et al. PI3K/Akt and apoptosis: size matters. Oncogene 2003;22:8983–98.

11. Fresno Vara JA, Casado E, de Castro J, et al. PI3K/Akt signalling pathway and cancer. Cancer Treat Rev 2004;30:193–204.
12. Davies H, Bignell GR, Cox C, et al. Mutations of the BRAF gene in human cancer. Nature 2002;417:949–54.
13. Mercer KE, Pritchard CA. Raf proteins and cancer: B-Raf is identified as a mutational target. Biochim Biophys Acta 2003;1653:25–40.
14. Markman B, Atzori F, Perez-Garcia J, et al. Status of PI3K inhibition and biomarker development in cancer therapeutics. Ann Oncol 2010;21:683–91.
15. Simpson L, Parsons R. PTEN: life as a tumor suppressor. Exp Cell Res 2001;264: 29–41.
16. Weng LP, Smith WM, Dahia PL, et al. PTEN suppresses breast cancer cell growth by phosphatase activity-dependent G1 arrest followed by cell death. Cancer Res 1999;59:5808–14.
17. Kanae Y, Endoh D, Yokota H, et al. Expression of the PTEN tumor suppressor gene in malignant mammary gland tumors of dogs. Am J Vet Res 2006;67:127–33.
18. Koenig A, Bianco SR, Fosmire S, et al. Expression and significance of p53, rb, p21/waf-1, p16/ink-4a, and PTEN tumor suppressors in canine melanoma. Vet Pathol 2002;39:458–72.
19. Levine RA, Forest T, Smith C. Tumor suppressor PTEN is mutated in canine osteosarcoma cell lines and tumors. Vet Pathol 2002;39:372–8.
20. London CA, Hannah AL, Zadovoskaya R, et al. Phase I dose-escalating study of SU11654, a small molecule receptor tyrosine kinase inhibitor, in dogs with spontaneous malignancies. Clin Cancer Res 2003;9:2755–68.
21. Yancey MF, Merritt DA, Lesman SP, et al. Pharmacokinetic properties of toceranib phosphate (Palladia, SU11654), a novel tyrosine kinase inhibitor, in laboratory dogs and dogs with mast cell tumors. J Vet Pharmacol Ther 2010;33: 162–71.
22. Yancey MF, Merritt DA, White JA, et al. Distribution, metabolism, and excretion of toceranib phosphate (Palladia, SU11654), a novel tyrosine kinase inhibitor, in dogs. J Vet Pharmacol Ther 2010;33:154–61.
23. Papaetis GS, Syrigos KN. Sunitinib: a multitargeted receptor tyrosine kinase inhibitor in the era of molecular cancer therapies. BioDrugs 2009;23:377–89.
24. London C, Mathie T, Stingle N, et al. Preliminary evidence for biologic activity of toceranib phosphate (Palladia) in solid tumours. Vet Comp Oncol 2012;10:194–205.
25. Marcinowska A, Warland J, Brearley M, et al. A novel approach to treatment of lymphangiosarcoma in a boxer dog. J Small Anim Pract 2013;54:334–7.
26. Perez ML, Culver S, Owen JL, et al. Partial cytogenetic response with toceranib and prednisone treatment in a young dog with chronic monocytic leukemia. Anticancer Drugs 2013;24:1098–103.
27. Chon E, McCartan L, Kubicek LN, et al. Safety evaluation of combination toceranib phosphate (Palladia(R)) and piroxicam in tumour-bearing dogs (excluding mast cell tumours): a phase I dose-finding study. Vet Comp Oncol 2012;10:184–93.
28. Robat C, London C, Bunting L, et al. Safety evaluation of combination vinblastine and toceranib phosphate (Palladia) in dogs: a phase I dose-finding study. Vet Comp Oncol 2012;10:174–83.
29. Carlsten KS, London CA, Haney S, et al. Multicenter prospective trial of hypofractionated radiation treatment, toceranib, and prednisone for measurable canine mast cell tumors. J Vet Intern Med 2012;26:135–41.
30. Burton JH, Mitchell L, Thamm DH, et al. Low-dose cyclophosphamide selectively decreases regulatory T cells and inhibits angiogenesis in dogs with soft tissue sarcoma. J Vet Intern Med 2011;25:920–6.

31. Ko JS, Zea AH, Rini BI, et al. Sunitinib mediates reversal of myeloid-derived suppressor cell accumulation in renal cell carcinoma patients. Clin Cancer Res 2009;15:2148–57.

32. Mitchell L, Thamm DH, Biller BJ. Clinical and immunomodulatory effects of toceranib combined with low-dose cyclophosphamide in dogs with cancer. J Vet Intern Med 2012;26:355–62.

33. Bernabe LF, Portela R, Nguyen S, et al. Evaluation of the adverse event profile and pharmacodynamics of toceranib phosphate administered to dogs with solid tumors at doses below the maximum tolerated dose. BMC Vet Res 2013;9:190.

34. Hahn KA, Legendre AM, Shaw NG, et al. Evaluation of 12- and 24-month survival rates after treatment with masitinib in dogs with nonresectable mast cell tumors. Am J Vet Res 2010;71:1354–61.

35. Smrkovski OA, Essick L, Rohrbach BW, et al. Masitinib mesylate for metastatic and non-resectable canine cutaneous mast cell tumours. Vet Comp Oncol 2013. [Epub ahead of print]. http://dx.doi.org/10.1111/vco.12053. PMID:23845124.

36. Isotani M, Ishida N, Tominaga M, et al. Effect of tyrosine kinase inhibition by imatinib mesylate on mast cell tumors in dogs. J Vet Intern Med 2008;22:985–8.

37. Marconato L, Bettini G, Giacoboni C, et al. Clinicopathological features and outcome for dogs with mast cell tumors and bone marrow involvement. J Vet Intern Med 2008;22:1001–7.

38. Yamada O, Kobayashi M, Sugisaki O, et al. Imatinib elicited a favorable response in a dog with a mast cell tumor carrying a c-kit c.1523A>T mutation via suppression of constitutive KIT activation. Vet Immunol Immunopathol 2011;142:101–6.

39. Isotani M, Tamura K, Yagihara H, et al. Identification of a c-kit exon 8 internal tandem duplication in a feline mast cell tumor case and its favorable response to the tyrosine kinase inhibitor imatinib mesylate. Vet Immunol Immunopathol 2006;114:168–72.

40. Isotani M, Yamada O, Lachowicz JL, et al. Mutations in the fifth immunoglobulin-like domain of kit are common and potentially sensitive to imatinib mesylate in feline mast cell tumours. Br J Haematol 2010;148:144–53.

41. Kobayashi M, Kuroki S, Ito K, et al. Imatinib-associated tumour response in a dog with a non-resectable gastrointestinal stromal tumour harbouring a c-kit exon 11 deletion mutation. Vet J 2013;198:271–4.

42. Pallotti MC, Pantaleo MA, Nannini M, et al. Development of a nephrotic syndrome in a patient with gastrointestinal stromal tumor during a long-time treatment with sunitinib. Case Rep Oncol 2012;5:651–6.

43. Patel TV, Morgan JA, Demetri GD, et al. A preeclampsia-like syndrome characterized by reversible hypertension and proteinuria induced by the multitargeted kinase inhibitors sunitinib and sorafenib. J Natl Cancer Inst 2008;100:282–4.

44. Turan N, Benekli M, Ozturk SC, et al. Sunitinib- and sorafenib-induced nephrotic syndrome in a patient with gastrointestinal stromal tumor. Ann Pharmacother 2012;46:e27.

45. Brown MR, Cianciolo RE, Nabity MB, et al. Masitinib-associated minimal change disease with acute tubular necrosis resulting in acute kidney injury in a dog. J Vet Intern Med 2013;27:1622–6.

46. Choi HK, Lee K. Recent updates on the development of ganetespib as a Hsp90 inhibitor. Arch Pharm Res 2012;35:1855–9.

47. London CA, Bear MD, McCleese J, et al. Phase I evaluation of STA-1474, a prodrug of the novel HSP90 inhibitor ganetespib, in dogs with spontaneous cancer. PLoS One 2011;6:e27018.

48. Xu D, Grishin NV, Chook YM. NESdb: a database of NES-containing CRM1 cargoes. Mol Biol Cell 2012;23:3673–6.
49. Daelemans D, Costes SV, Lockett S, et al. Kinetic and molecular analysis of nuclear export factor CRM1 association with its cargo in vivo. Mol Cell Biol 2005;25:728–39.
50. Fornerod M, Ohno M, Yoshida M, et al. CRM1 is an export receptor for leucine-rich nuclear export signals. Cell 1997;90:1051–60.
51. Nguyen KT, Holloway MP, Altura RA. The CRM1 nuclear export protein in normal development and disease. Int J Biochem Mol Biol 2012;3:137–51.
52. Turner JG, Dawson J, Sullivan DM. Nuclear export of proteins and drug resistance in cancer. Biochem Pharmacol 2012;83:1021–32.
53. Turner JG, Sullivan DM. CRM1-mediated nuclear export of proteins and drug resistance in cancer. Curr Med Chem 2008;15:2648–55.
54. Azmi AS, Aboukameel A, Bao B, et al. Selective inhibitors of nuclear export block pancreatic cancer cell proliferation and reduce tumor growth in mice. Gastroenterology 2013;144:447–56.
55. McCauley D, Landesman Y, Senapedis W, et al. Preclinical evaluation of selective inhibitors of nuclear export (SINE) in basal-like breast cancer (BLBC). J Clin Oncol 2012;30(Suppl) [abstract: 1055].
56. Lapalombella R, Sun Q, Williams K, et al. Selective inhibitors of nuclear export show that CRM1/XPO1 is a target in chronic lymphocytic leukemia. Blood 2012;120:4621–34.
57. Etchin J, Sun Q, Kentsis A, et al. Antileukemic activity of nuclear export inhibitors that spare normal hematopoietic cells. Leukemia 2013;27:66–74.
58. Kenward MG, Roger JH. Small sample inference for fixed effects from restricted maximum likelihood. Biometrics 1997;53:983–97.
59. Ropero S, Esteller M. The role of histone deacetylases (HDACs) in human cancer. Mol Oncol 2007;1:19–25.
60. Feinberg AP, Tycko B. The history of cancer epigenetics. Nat Rev Cancer 2004; 4:143–53.
61. Zhu P, Martin E, Mengwasser J, et al. Induction of HDAC2 expression upon loss of APC in colorectal tumorigenesis. Cancer Cell 2004;5:455–63.
62. Marchion DC, Bicaku E, Daud AI, et al. In vivo synergy between topoisomerase II and histone deacetylase inhibitors: predictive correlates. Mol Cancer Ther 2005;4:1993–2000.
63. Munster P, Marchion D, Bicaku E, et al. Clinical and biological effects of valproic acid as a histone deacetylase inhibitor on tumor and surrogate tissues: phase I/II trial of valproic acid and epirubicin/FEC. Clin Cancer Res 2009;15:2488–96.
64. Munster P, Marchion D, Bicaku E, et al. Phase I trial of histone deacetylase inhibition by valproic acid followed by the topoisomerase II inhibitor epirubicin in advanced solid tumors: a clinical and translational study. J Clin Oncol 2007;25:1979–85.
65. Wittenburg LA, Bisson L, Rose BJ, et al. The histone deacetylase inhibitor valproic acid sensitizes human and canine osteosarcoma to doxorubicin. Cancer Chemother Pharmacol 2011;67:83–92.
66. Wittenburg LA, Gustafson DL, Thamm DH. Phase I pharmacokinetic and pharmacodynamic evaluation of combined valproic acid/doxorubicin treatment in dogs with spontaneous cancer. Clin Cancer Res 2010;16:4832–42.
67. Rosenzweig SA. Acquired resistance to drugs targeting receptor tyrosine kinases. Biochem Pharmacol 2012;83:1041–8.
68. O'Hare T, Eide CA, Deininger MW. Bcr-Abl kinase domain mutations, drug resistance, and the road to a cure for chronic myeloid leukemia. Blood 2007;110: 2242–9.

69. O'Hare T, Eide CA, Deininger MW. Bcr-Abl kinase domain mutations and the unsettled problem of Bcr-AblT315I: looking into the future of controlling drug resistance in chronic myeloid leukemia. Clin Lymphoma Myeloma 2007;7(Suppl 3): S120–30.
70. Mahon FX, Deininger MW, Schultheis B, et al. Selection and characterization of BCR-ABL positive cell lines with differential sensitivity to the tyrosine kinase inhibitor STI571: diverse mechanisms of resistance. Blood 2000;96:1070–9.
71. Kosaka T, Yamaki E, Mogi A, et al. Mechanisms of resistance to EGFR TKIs and development of a new generation of drugs in non-small-cell lung cancer. J Biomed Biotechnol 2011;2011:165214.

Advances in Veterinary Radiation Therapy

Targeting Tumors and Improving Patient Comfort

Susan M. LaRue, DVM, PhD*, James T. Custis, DVM, MS

KEYWORDS

- Veterinary radiation therapy • Intensity-modulated radiation therapy
- Stereotactic radiation therapy • Image-guided radiation therapy

KEY POINTS

- Newer technology, such as intensity-modulated radiation therapy (IMRT), can dramatically decrease acute radiation side effects, making patients much more comfortable during and after treatment.
- Stereotactic radiation therapy (SRT) for definitive treatment can be delivered in 1 to 5 fractions, with minimal radiation-associated effects.
- Image-guided radiation therapy can be used to direct treatment in locations previously not amenable to radiation therapy.
- Traditional fractionated radiation therapy remains the most commonly available type of radiation therapy in veterinary medicine and is the standard of care for many tumors. Improved pain management plans help improve patient comfort.

INTRODUCTION

A remarkable transformation has occurred over the past 20 years in the management of human cancers (**Fig. 1**). The ability to diagnose, stage, and monitor disease has been enhanced by advances in imaging, including positron emission tomography–computed tomography (PET-CT). Advances in radiation planning and dose delivery, including intensity-modulated radiation therapy (IMRT), allows dose to be "painted" onto the tumor while sparing surrounding normal tissues. IMRT has improved tumor control for many types of cancer in people, including prostate cancer and head and neck cancers, while vastly decreasing radiation-associated side effects. Stereotactic radiation therapy (SRT), which can be delivered via gamma knife, cyber knife, or linear

Funding Sources: Varian Medical Systems YC VA05, Palo Alto, CA; Morris Animal Foundation D09FE-003, D10FE-405 (S.M. LaRue); Dani Foundation; Varian Medical Systems, Palo Alto, CA (J.T. Custis).
Department of Environmental and Radiological Health Sciences, Colorado State University Flint Animal Cancer Center, 300 West Drake Road, Fort Collins, CO 80523, USA
* Corresponding author.
E-mail address: slarue@colostate.edu

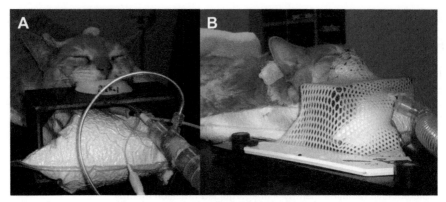

Fig. 1. (A) Cat positioned with a vacu-lock pillow and bite block that is pegged into a carbon fiber platform that is indexed to the CT and radiation therapy couches. (B) An acrylic face mask is secured over the face and platform.

accelerators with image guidance, has surged into cancer care. Definitive treatment with SRT can be delivered in 1 to 5 treatments for some types of cancers. Now these technologies are available in veterinary medicine. This article discusses the role of these advancements in the treatment of veterinary patients with cancer and reviews more traditional radiation treatment.

RADIATION ONCOLOGY IN VETERINARY MEDICINE: PAST TO PRESENT

Life expectancy for pet animals has increased, and cancer is primarily a disease of aging populations. As such, the prevalence of cancer in pet animals is increasing, and cancer is thought to be the leading cause of death in older dogs. With the increased interest from clients and veterinarians in the diagnosis and treatment of pet animals with cancer, veterinary oncology has become a vital discipline. Stephen Withrow and other early oncologists were instrumental in changing prevailing attitudes about treating pets with cancer.[1] Veterinary medical oncology was conferred specialty status within the American College of Veterinary Internal medicine in 1988, and there are currently more than 370 diplomates, who are trained in the diagnosis, staging, and management of cancer, including chemotherapy treatment. Oncologic surgery is now a recognized subspecialty in the American College of Veterinary Surgeons, requiring an additional year of fellowship training directed specifically at cancer treatment. In 1994, veterinary radiation oncology was recognized as a specialty within the American College of Veterinary Radiology. Currently there are more than 90 board-certified radiation oncologists, and more than 60 facilities in the United States and Canada. Radiation oncology also is available in Europe, Asia, and South America. Integration of surgical oncology, medical oncology, and radiation oncology provides optimal treatment outcome, regardless of species.

Surprisingly, despite limited availability, radiation therapy was the first commonly reported therapy for animal patients with cancer. Reports describing the treatment of canine cancers were published soon after the discovery of radiation by Roentgen.[2,3] Alois Pommer, a veterinarian from Austria, investigated normal tissue responses in the 1930s, and then reported outcomes from systematic treatment of more than 1000 animals.[4,5] His publications were outcome based and provided information regarding tumor control and adverse radiation effects. He developed the first commonly used veterinary protocol, 4 Gy delivered on Monday, Wednesday, and

Friday for 10 to 12 treatments. Although we now recognize that this protocol is far from optimal, it was established based on practicality and good clinical observation. He treated every other day because no available anesthesia agents could be safely administered on a daily basis so he used slings and other restraining devices. He inferred from his data that cells in mitosis may be more sensitive to radiation, and so fractionation (splitting the dose into multiple smaller treatments) improved the probability of radiation affecting more cells at this sensitive time. He recognized that treating over a relatively short time period could benefit rapidly growing tumors.

After safer anesthetic agents were developed, many veterinary radiation facilities began treating on a daily basis, but treatment duration was still restricted in length, or accelerated, compared with human protocols. Interestingly, human radiation oncologists are prescribing accelerated protocols more frequently to help combat the problem of accelerated repopulation (an increase in tumor cell growth) that occurs when tumors are treated over a period longer than 4 weeks.[6] Clearly, the similarities between human tumors and animal tumors, including response to radiation treatment, have been recognized.

In 1938, the University of Pennsylvania became the first veterinary school to acquire orthovoltage radiation therapy equipment for the treatment of animal patients.[7] Dr M.A. Emmerson, head of the department of radiology at the veterinary school, went to Vienna to study with Pommer.[8] When he returned, he treated more than 1000 animals, including horses, ponies, cows, goats, dogs, cats, and rats during the first 18 months.[9]

Much has been learned from animal patients with cancer that has benefited not only animals but humans as well.[10] By the late 1970s, Edward L. Gillette, a radiation oncologist with advanced training in radiation biology, established a comparative oncology program at Colorado State University.[11,12] His program received early NIH funding for translational research. Translational research by Gillette, Donald Thrall, Mark Dewhirst, and Patrick Gavin not only solidified the value of the pet tumor model, but also established radiation therapy as the standard for care for many pet animal tumors.[13–17]

BIOLOGICAL PRINCIPLES AND TECHNICAL ADVANCES

The biological principles and the technological developments are the same for human and veterinary radiation oncology and are discussed in tandem. Orthovoltage therapy machines were the first widely used form of external-beam radiation therapy, but have limitations. X-rays produced by orthovoltage therapy units have low energy and lack tissue penetration. The dose to skin is higher than the prescribed tumor dose, leading to severe acute effects to skin. Dose is highly dependent on the proton number of the tissue, leading to an uneven and unpredictable dose distribution (eg, bone receives a much higher dose than adjacent soft tissue structures). Despite these technical liabilities, Henri Coutard,[18,19] a radiation oncologist at the Pierre and Marie Curie Institute in Paris, identified a number of important radiation oncology principles that hold true today. He recognized that at a comparable dose, larger radiation fields were associated with a greater percentage of adverse late effects. He found that when dose was delivered in small "fractions" the normal tissues tolerated a higher radiation dose. He observed that if the duration of time over which radiation treatment was extended, tumor control was compromised. Pommer,[4,5] on the veterinary side, was doing similar work evaluating response to treatment. Orthovoltage was the primary mode of radiation therapy in veterinary medicine until the 1980s. Superficial tumors in human and veterinary medicine are still treated with orthovoltage therapy on a limited basis.

The Introduction of Megavoltage Radiation Therapy

Technical advances associated with World War II led to the development of cobalt radiation therapy and high-energy linear accelerators. Cobalt machines house a radioactive cobalt source that produces high-energy gamma rays. Accelerators produce x-rays by accelerating electrons into a gold or tungsten target, producing high-energy x-rays. X-rays and gamma rays with energy over a million electron volts are referred to as megavoltage radiation. Unlike orthovoltage radiation, this megavoltage radiation spares skin and has greater depth of penetration. Perhaps more importantly, radiation dose is evenly distributed through tissues and can be accurately predicted. Point-dose calculations and 3-dimensional conformal radiation therapy (3D-CRT) are based on the predictability of dose distribution. There is no significant biological difference between the photons produced by cobalt radiation therapy machines and linear accelerators. Both systems can be used for manual point-dose calculations and for 3D-CRT radiation planning. However, accelerators can be adapted to produce electrons of various energies to treat superficial tumors, and some accelerators can produce more than one photon energy, although 6 MV is the most common photon energy used in veterinary medicine. Newer accelerators also may have technology that can provide IMRT and SRT. Linear accelerators now dominate radiation therapy in both human and veterinary medicine.

Manual Point-Dose Calculations

Delivering radiation treatment using 2 parallel opposed beams is based on manual calculation of reference in the tissues. This strategy can provide an even dose through the tissues when treating cubic or rectangular prismlike structures, where the dose to the treatment field can be predicted accurately by dose to the reference point. However, dose to the planning target volume (PTV) can be overestimated or underestimated based on the size of the patient relative to the energy of the photons. In veterinary radiation oncology, this approach remains the standard of care for incompletely excised soft tissue sarcomas and mast cell tumors of the extremities.[20,21] Treatment outcome is outstanding and it is unlikely that newer technologies, such as IMRT, can improve tumor control. Unfortunately, this treatment can be associated with severe acute radiation effects to the skin. These include erythema, dry desquamation, and moist desquamation. Improved pain control protocols can keep these patients comfortable. The area should be kept clean, but not scrubbed. Prevention of self-mutilation is important, and bandaging and/or Elizabethan or bite-not collars may be required to keep the area unperturbed.

Manual dose calculation is not reliant on CT-based or magnetic resonance imaging (MRI)-based imaging, making the treatment less costly. Manual point dose calculations also are useful for tumors of the spine, mediastinum, and whole/partial brain treatment; these regions of the body also have relatively uniform depth. This method is used successfully to palliate a wide variety of tumors in a number of locations.[22,23]

Electron therapy is a form of external-beam radiation therapy in which electrons are directed at the tumor. Many linear accelerators are equipped to provide electron therapy in addition to photon therapy and will include a range of electron energies. Electrons do not penetrate as well as x-rays, which are normally used for external-beam radiation therapy, and once they reach their maximum dose, the dose falls off dramatically. They are particularly useful for treatment of skin tumors over the abdomen, so that excess radiation does not reach the intestinal tract, and for tumors over the thorax, so that the dose of radiation to the lungs can be limited. Electrons also are useful for tumors near the eye. A special ceramic-covered tungsten contact lens block can be placed over the eye to greatly diminish dose, while the prescribed dose can be delivered to the area surrounding the eye. Point-dose calculations are generally used for electron beam therapy, although computerized planning systems for electrons also are available.

3D-CRT

The 3D-CRT uses CT-based imaging to generate 3D images of specific internal structures. Both tumor and normal tissue structures are identified by the radiation oncologist and are individually labeled, or "contoured," so the planning system can recognize the structures. The planning system can then relate information about radiation dose to the specific structures of interest. The gross tumor volume (GTV) includes only gross tumor, whereas the clinical target volume (CTV) also includes a margin so that microscopic disease can be included. CTV expansions are based on the known behavior of the tumor. For example, the CTV expansion would be larger for a sarcoma, where microscopic disease may be located centimeters from the gross disease, than for a carcinoma, where microscopic disease does not extend as far. The resulting dose volume histogram (DVH) provides a precise description of the prescribed dose to the tumor and to critical normal tissue structures. Customized cerobend blocks or static multileaf collimators are used to exclude normal tissue structures that do not overlie the tumor. An important but sometimes overlooked aspect of 3D-CRT is the use of positioning devices, such as face masks and vacu-lock positioning bags to allow precise repositioning from fraction to fraction (**Fig. 1**). With confirmation by a radiation medical physicist, these types of positioning devices can decrease PTV (planning target volume) expansion. The PTV expansion takes the imprecision of the patient positioning into account. With better immobilization, a smaller PTV expansion can be applied, limiting the radiation dose to normal surrounding tissues. The 3D-CRT is the standard of care in radiation therapy for many cancers treated in veterinary medicine, particularly oral tumors and brain tumors. It also has been used for the treatment of intranasal tumors; however, it is associated with substantial acute radiation effects, such as mucositis, dermatitis, and keratitis. Newer modalities, such as IMRT, that limit radiation effects to the skin and mucous membranes provide greater patient comfort, although improvement in disease-free interval or survival has not been demonstrated. The 3D-CRT also remains standard of care for a number of human cancers, including breast cancer and lung cancers.

IMRT

IMRT resulted from advancements in radiation treatment planning. Sophisticated computer algorithms led to what is known as inverse treatment planning. Inverse planning requires that the various tumor structures (GTV, CTV, and PTV), as well as critical normal tissue structures be identified and contoured into the planning system. Optimization objectives for each structure are entered, and dose objectives and normal tissue constraints are defined. In general, these plans require from 5 to 12 radiation fields. But instead of each field being static, the multileaf collimator moves during treatment (either with sliding leaf or step-and-shoot technology), providing many degrees of freedom for the planning algorithm. This technology is valuable for treating geometrically complex tumors in animals, such as brain, intranasal, vertebral body, bladder, prostate, and perineal tumors. IMRT is standard of care for the treatment of prostate tumors, head and neck cancers, vertebral cancers, some brain cancers, and pelvic cancers in humans. There are 2 major benefits associated with IMRT. First, dose to adjacent normal tissue structures can be minimized, dramatically reducing acute effects. Second, dose can be increased because dose to late-responding tissues can be minimized, leading to improved tumor control. In the treatment of human prostatic cancers, acute effects were minimized despite dose escalation, which led to superior tumor control. **Fig. 2**A–C show the GTV (red line), CTV (green line), and PTV (shaded green) of a large feline pituitary tumor. **Fig. 2**D is the dose volume histogram where the CTV for 3D-CRT and IMRT have been normalized. So, with the same dose to tumor structures, the dose to normal brain is greatly reduced in the IMRT plan. This technology has been shown to markedly decrease radiation acute effects associated with the treatment of canine nasal tumors.[24,25] Improvement in survival has not been documented; however, published reports did not escalate radiation dose.[24,25] IMRT combined with dose escalation could be an important tool to improve outcome for a number of canine and feline tumors.

Advanced Imaging for Better Tumor Localization During Planning

With the development of IMRT, determining tumor location became more critical because dose could now be accurately delivered, or painted, onto the tumor. Going from the cubical dose distributions of 3D-CRT to the sculpted doses of IMRT left little room for error in contouring. Imaging technology advanced to allow for the fusion of CT and MR scans, superimposing the images. This merged the boney definition from the CT scan with the soft tissue information from the MRI. This is particularly important for brain tumors, because some tumors are not visible on CT scans. For optimal fusion, the MRI sequences most relevant to planning (T1 pre, T2 and T1

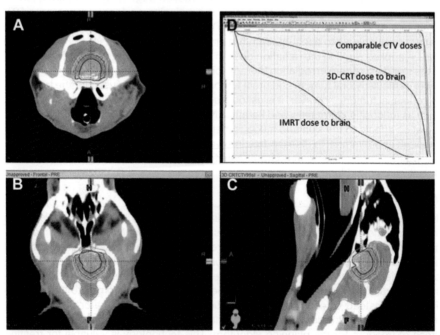

Fig. 2. (A–C) The axial, coronal, and sagittal sections of a large feline pituitary tumor. The red line shows the GTV, the green line the CTV, and the shaded green the PTV. (D) A dose-volume histogram comparing the 3D-CRT and IMRT plans that have been normalized so that that 95% of the CTV dose is administered to 95% of the CTV volume (*green lines*). The red line with squares shows the DVH of dose to brain from the 3D-CRT plan, whereas the red line with squares shows the dose to brain from the IMRT plan. The brain receives less dose using IMRT. ([D] *Courtesy of* Yoshikawa H, DVM, PhD, Nara, Japan.)

post) should be obtained using the same slice thickness of the CT scan. Most radiation oncologists use 2-mm scanning thickness for planning. **Fig. 3** shows a CT scan, where the tumor is not visible, the fused CT/MRI with the GTV drawn in red, and the MRI, showing the tumor.

PET-CT imaging became available in the 1990s. PET-CT combines important metabolic information from PET with the detailed anatomic information from the CT scan. PET is a type of nuclear medicine in which positrons from an injected radioisotope combine with nearby electrons, resulting in 2 coincident 511-keV photons that are detected by a ring of detectors in the scanner. The most commonly used isotope for PET-CT is 2-^{18}F-Fluoro-2-Deoxy-D-Glucose (^{18}F-FDG), a glucose analog radiotracer that accumulates in areas with high glucose uptake and high cellular metabolism. A tumor's affinity for glucose is exploited, so metabolically active areas will be detected. The functional information from the PET is merged with a CT, obtained with the patient in the same position, thus providing anatomic definition to the metabolic information. PET-CT is now commonly used in human cancer facilities for staging, radiation planning, and to determine chemotherapy or chemo-radiation response.[26] PET and PET-CT have become more recently available in veterinary medicine. For radiation therapy planning, PET-CT helps define diffuse tumors located in soft tissue structures and near mucous membranes. Twelve cats with oral squamous cell carcinomas underwent ^{18}F-FDG PET-CT before radiation planning. All tumors were FDG avid and apparent on ^{18}F-FDG images. Soft tissue tumors in the lingual/laryngeal tumors that were poorly defined on CT were highly visible and more extensive on ^{18}F-FDG PET-CT (**Fig. 4**).[27,28]

^{18}F-FDT PET-CT also was found to be an important tool for staging cats with squamous cell carcinoma.[28] Randall and colleagues[28] identified lymph node involvement and metastatic disease undetected by routine staging. Work is ongoing evaluating different radionuclides that can also be used to look for different end points. ^{64}Cu-diacetyl-bis(N4-methylsemicarbazone) is being evaluated as a marker of tumor hypoxia.[29] Sodium fluoride F[18] is being evaluated as a marker for boney metastasis and other boney disorders.[30]

Image-Guided Radiation Therapy

Newer linear accelerators can be equipped with on-board imaging (OBI). Although OBI is essential for stereotactic radiation therapy, it also can be useful for IMRT and dynamic adaptive radiation therapy (DART). Image-guided intensity-modulated radiation therapy was used to treat 19 dogs with bladder and/or prostate cancer. This technique decreases the PTV expansion required to account for the day-to-day movement of the

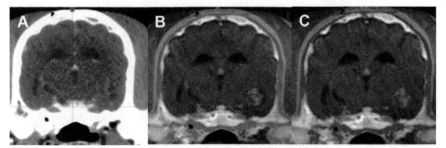

Fig. 3. (*A*) A CT scan of brain with minimal evidence of tumor. (*B*) A fused MRI/CT with the tumor GTV outlined in red. (*C*) A T1 post-gadolinium contrast study, where the tumor is evident. ([C] *Courtesy of* Yoshikawa H, DVM, PhD, Nara, Japan.)

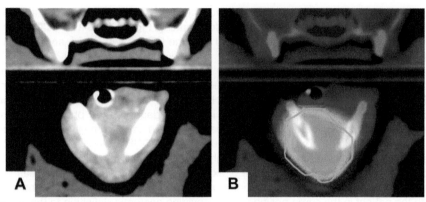

Fig. 4. (*A*) A CT from a cat with a sublingual squamous cell carcinoma. The tumor cannot be identified. (*B*) The PET-CT from the same patient. Tumor volume can be readily identified. ([*B*] *From* Yoshikawa H, Randall EK, Kraft SL, et al. Comparison between 2-(18) F-Fluoro-2-Deoxy-D-glucose positron emission tomography and contrast-enhanced computed tomography for measuring gross tumor volume in cats with oral squamous cell carcinoma. Vet Radiol Ultrasound 2013;54:313; with permission.)

bladder and colon.[31] A cone-beam CT (CBCT), which is part of the OBI system, was acquired before each treatment and the field could be adjusted to include the PTV. Median survival of dogs in the study was more than 600 days, far surpassing previous reports. The treatment was well tolerated by the patients, with minimal gastrointestinal side effects and owners had a high level of satisfaction for the overall treatment experience.[32] **Fig. 5** shows the dose distribution to the bladder and surrounding normal tissue structures that is obtained using image-guided intensity-modulated radiotherapy (IGIMRT). Minimal dose is delivered to the colon and small intestines.

DART

DART is a technique in which the radiation plan is adapted as the tumor shrinks during treatment. This technique requires on-board image guidance. The CBCT

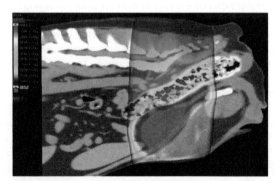

Fig. 5. A typical dose-distribution for IMIGRT, depicted as a color-wash superimposed over the simulation CT. A steep dose gradient between target volumes and organs at risk is shown with areas of relatively high dose in red and orange, and lower doses in yellow, green, and blue. Note that dose to colon and small intestine is considerably lower than the tumor dose. (*From* Nolan MW, Kogan L, Griffin LR, et al. Intensity-modulated and image-guided radiation therapy for treatment of genitourinary carcinomas in dogs. J Vet Intern Med 2012;26(4):987–95; with permission.)

data acquired at treatment can be uploaded into the treatment-planning system, and adjustments (real-time or before the next treatment) to the treatment plan can be made. This is important when the tumor has substantial shrinkage during treatment. **Fig. 6** shows that the original location of the left eye has moved during therapy, and without planning adjustment, the eye would have received unnecessary dose. **Fig. 6**B shows the adjustment. DART is frequently used for IGIMRT and for the treatment of rapidly responding tumors such as lymphoma. DART can be used for IMRT and SRT, however the overall treatment time of SRT is usually so short that significant shrinkage has not yet occurred.

SRT

A number of terms are used to describe this nonsurgical radiation therapy technique. Stereotactic radiosurgery (SRS) refers primarily to treatment of brain tumors and is generally administered in one fraction. SRT, stereotactic body radiation therapy, and stereotactic ablative radiation therapy are all terms used to describe hypofractionated treatment administered in 2 to 5 fractions. SRT will be used generically in this article. SRT is highly focused radiation that relies on a steep dose gradient between the tumor and surrounding normal tissue structures. It therefore requires some sort of stereotactic imaging system to confirm fiducial location. SRT requires a macroscopic tumor target, so it is not useful for treating microscopic disease that remains after surgical excision. SRS generally (but not always) refers a single treatment and

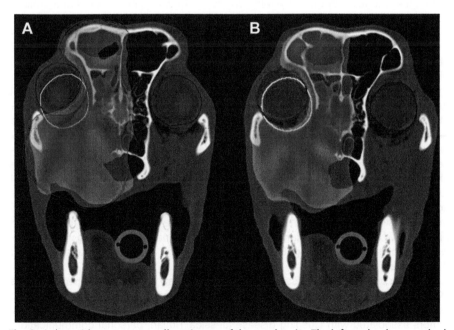

Fig. 6. A dog with a squamous cell carcinoma of the nasal cavity. The left eye has been pushed out of normal position by the tumor. (*A*) A dose colorwash, with the prescribed dose shown in orange to red. The original position of the eye is outlined in blue, but during treatment the tumor shrank and the eye returned to a more normal position (*yellow outline*). If the plan had not been modified, the eye would have received unnecessary dose. (*B*) A DART adaptation that recognizes and adjusts dose for the positional change of the eye.

is most commonly used for brain lesions. The gamma knife, developed by Lars Leksell, was the first device developed for SRS administration.[33] Still in use, it was designed for brain cancers and required a frame-based system screwed into the skull. The gamma knife has 201 cobalt sources that can be directed toward a single target. By the 1990s, stereotactic imaging had made technological advances and other systems became available that were more conducive to administering more than one fraction. For tumors not located near radiation-sensitive structures, single fraction (SRS) may have radiobiological advantages; however, for tumors near radiation-sensitive structures, such as spinal cord, rectum, and optic chiasm, coarsely fractionating the radiation may be advantageous to help spare these structures. SRT is undergoing widespread evaluation in human clinical trials and has become the standard-of-care treatment for a number of tumors.[34–36] Forward planning and inverse planning systems can both be used for SRT, depending on the system. Beams can be positioned in coplanar or noncoplanar angles. Having positional verification allows for minimal PTV expansion, which decreases radiation acute effects.

A number of different systems have been developed for SRT. The body gamma knife is an adaptation of the original gamma knife, but can be positioned around many more parts of the body. The cyberknife is a robotic radiosurgery system.[37] The robotic arm directs a small linear accelerator beam. A radiofrequency imaging system identifies implanted fiducial markers to ensure accuracy. Accelerator-based systems, such as the Varian Trilogy (Palo Alto, California), have OBI systems including both kilovolt radiographs and CBCT, so patient positioning can be verified before treatment. All of these systems are accurate and there are pros and cons to each system. The cyberknife may provide better dose distributions to small tumors, but accelerator-based systems can treat regional nodes in addition to the primary tumor, and administration is faster. Good SRT, regardless of administrating device, still relies on good treatment planning and input from the radiation oncologist and physicist.

In veterinary medicine, SRS or SRT for bone tumors has provided excellent local tumor control, providing a nonsurgical limb-sparing option.[38,39] The structural integrity of the bone needs to be evaluated before treatment. Extremely lytic tumors are associated with early fracture.[40] Like patients with osteosarcoma treated with amputation, patient survival is still limited by the development of metastatic disease. Patients receiving SRT limb sparing should have concomitant or adjunctive chemotherapy to help address distant spread. SRT delivered in 3 fractions for nasal tumors provides tumor control comparable to that obtained with fractionated radiation protocols with minimal acute radiation effects.[41] For presumed meningiomas, median survival is more than 550 days, comparable to fractionated protocols.[42] **Fig. 7** shows a CT image of a large sarcoma of the sinonasal cavity along with a color-wash of dose distribution. **Fig. 8** shows the wolf-hybrid at the time of treatment and 2 years later.

Cats with pituitary tumors associated with acromegaly have 85% survival at 3 years (Kathryn Lunn, personal communication, 2014), with almost every cat having improved response to insulin.[43] However, the response is not as good for dogs with pituitary tumors associated with Cushing disease (Jessica Timian, personal communication, 2014), and traditional fractionated protocols are recommended. SRT also is useful for the treatment of many tumors that are not surgically resectable. Tumors of the pelvis, ribs, vertebra, thyroid, and heart have been safely treated and patient recovery time is minimal.

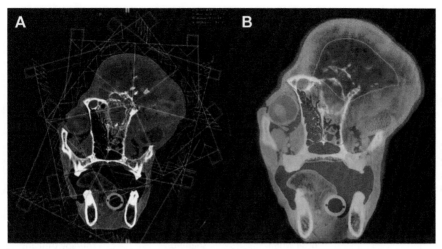

Fig. 7. (*A*) A CT scan of a sinomaxillary tumor, with beam positions used for the treatment plan. (*B*) A colorwash of the dose distribution, with prescribed dose in orange.

FUTURE DIRECTIONS

Radiation oncology has undergone important technical advancements over the past 20 years. Veterinary patients with cancer can benefit greatly as this technology becomes increasingly available. It is important to remember that these new technologies add to our arsenal of treatment options, and for many conditions older technologies still offer advantages (**Table 1**). The future holds the exciting promise of using PET-CT for improved staging and to identify areas of tumor hypoxia for dose escalation. The power of SRT is still being revealed. Optimization of SRT protocols, and combining with radiation sensitizers or other modifiers can lead to improved outcome. Veterinary medicine benefits greatly from scholarly work in human radiation oncology, and the spontaneously occurring canine and feline tumor models provide a tool for better understanding of radiation response in all species.

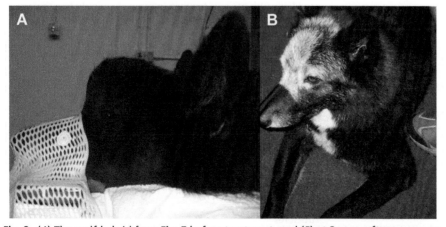

Fig. 8. (*A*) The wolf-hybrid from **Fig. 7** before treatment, and (*B*) at 2 years after treatment.

Table 1
Pros and cons of different radiation modalities

Technology	Advantages	Disadvantages	Useful For
Manual point calculation (parallel opposed portals)	Because advanced imaging is not required, can be less expensive	Dose to only 1 point is known, so can lead to overdosing or underdosing	Fractionated radiation therapy of microscopic disease of the extremities.
	Minimal time delay for treatment planning	Uneven distribution of dose when treating complex shapes	Tumors of rostral maxilla and mandible
	Can be used to treat microscopic disease		Can be used for brain and spine, but other options better.
	Even distribution of dose when treating cuboid structures using parallel opposed portals	No dose painting or shaping	Palliative radiation therapy of many sites
	Can use blocks or multileaf collimators to block dose to normal tissue structures if not overlying tumor		
Electrons	Limited penetration with rapid dose drop-off	Dose most predictable on flat surfaces.	Tumors or tumor beds over thorax and abdomen
			Tumors near eyelids where a protective shield can protect eye
3D-CRT	Can use beam modifiers, such as wedges, to alter dose distribution. Made possible by advanced imaging and treatment planning	Advanced imaging required (more expensive)	Fractionated radiation therapy of brain and spine/spinal cord tumors, pelvic tumors, mediastinal and heart-based tumors, head and neck tumors
	Can use glancing fields and multiple beams	No dose painting or shaping	Palliative radiation therapy of many sites
	Can obtain a dose volume histogram to better assess dose to tumor and normal tissue structures		

(continued on next page)

Table 1
(continued)

Technology	Advantages	Disadvantages	Useful For
IMRT	Able to better spare normal tissue structures, minimizing radiation effects Can use to treat gross or microscopic disease Dose escalation could lead to improved tumor control	Requires advanced accelerator, inverse treatment planning and record and verify technology	Nasal tumors, oral tumors, brain tumors, body wall tumors, urinary tract tumors
IGIMRT	Can treat tumors that move relative to bony anatomy, such as bladder and prostate tumors	Requires advanced equipment, including technology to verify tumor location before treatment	Canine bladder, prostate and urethral tumors; abdominal or thoracic wall tumors
SRT	Treatment completed in 1–5 fractions Minimal acute radiation effects	Requires advanced equipment including technology to verify tumor location prior to treatment. Do not use to treat canine pituitary tumors Cannot treat microscopic disease	Feline pituitary tumors, meningiomas, nasal tumors, bone tumors, thyroid tumors, lung tumors, mediastinal tumors, heart-based tumors, pelvic tumors Good for durable palliation at almost any site

Abbreviations: IGIMRT, image-guided intensity-modulated radiotherapy; IMRT, intensity-modulated radiotherapy; SRT, stereotactic radiation therapy; 3D-CRT, 3-dimensional conformal radiation therapy.

REFERENCES

1. Withrow SJ, Hirsch VM. Owner response to amputation of a pet's leg. Vet Med Small Anim Clin 1979;74(3):332, 334.
2. Eberlein R. Ein Versuch mit Roentgen'schen Strahlen. Monatsheftu praktischa Tierhailkunda. 1896. p. 7.
3. Eberlein R. Rontgentherapie bei Haustieren Verh Beirichte II. Hamburg: Rontgenkongr; 1906.
4. Pommer A, Maiolino A. Roentgen epilation and erythema doses of the skin in the dog. North Am Vet 1937;18:39–58.
5. Pommer A. X-ray therapy in veterinary medicine. In: Brandly CA, Jungher EL, editors. Advances in veterinary science. New York: Academic Press; 1958. p. 98–136.
6. Withers HR, Taylor JM, Maciejewski B. The hazard of accelerated tumor clonogen repopulation during radiotherapy. Acta Oncol 1988;27:131–46.
7. Emmerson MA. Veterinary x-ray therapy. Lederle veterinary bulletin, vol. 9. 1940. p. 3–8.
8. Gillette EL. History of veterinary radiation oncology. Vet Clin North Am Small Anim Pract 1997;27:1–6.
9. Emmerson MA. Veterinary X-ray Therapy, Lederle Veterinary Bulletin 1940;9.

10. Prier JE, Brodey RS. Canine neoplasia. A prototype for human cancer study. Bull World Health Organ 1963;29:331–44.
11. Gillette EL. Spontaneous canine neoplasms as models for therapeutic agents. In: Design of models for testing cancer therapeutic agents. 1982. p. 185–92.
12. Gillette EL. Veterinary radiotherapy. J Am Vet Med Assoc 1970;157:1707–12.
13. Gillette EL, McChesney SL, Dewhirst MW, et al. Response of canine oral carcinomas to heat and radiation. Int J Radiat Oncol Biol Phys 1987;13:1861–7.
14. Dewhirst MW, Connor WG, Sim DA. Preliminary results of a phase III trial of spontaneous animal tumors to heat and/or radiation: early normal tissue response and tumor volume influence on initial response. Int J Radiat Oncol Biol Phys 1982;8: 1951–61.
15. Thrall DE, Adams WM. Radiotherapy of squamous cell carcinomas of the canine nasal plane. Veterinary Radiology 1982;23(5):193–6.
16. Thrall DE. Orthovoltage radiotherapy of oral fibrosarcomas in dogs. J Am Vet Med Assoc 1981;179:159–62.
17. Gavin PR, Gillette EL. Radiation response of the canine cardiovascular system. Radiat Res 1982;90:489–500.
18. Coutard H. The results and methods of treatment of cancer by radiation. Ann Surg 1937;106:584–98.
19. Coutard H. Roentgen therapy of epitheliomas of the tonsillar region, hypopharynx larynx from 1920 to 1926. Am J Roentgenol 1932;28:313–31.
20. Gillette SM, Dewhirst MW, Gillette EL, et al. Response of canine soft tissue sarcomas to radiation or radiation plus hyperthermia: a randomized phase II study. Int J Hyperthermia 1992;8:309–20.
21. Frimberger AE, Moore AS, LaRue SM, et al. Radiotherapy of incompletely resected, moderately differentiated mast cell tumors in the dog: 37 cases (1989-1993). J Am Anim Hosp Assoc 1997;33:320–4.
22. Ramirez O III, Dodge RK, Page RL, et al. Palliative radiotherapy of appendicular osteosarcoma in 95 dogs. Vet Radiol Ultrasound 1999;40:517–22.
23. Carlsten KS, London CA, Haney S, et al. Multicenter prospective trial of hypofractionated radiation treatment, toceranib, and prednisone for measurable canine mast cell tumors. J Vet Intern Med 2012;26:135–41.
24. Hunley DW, Mauldin GN, Shiomitsu K, et al. Clinical outcome in dogs with nasal tumors treated with intensity-modulated radiation therapy. Can Vet J 2010;51: 293–300.
25. Lawrence JA, Forrest LJ, Turek MM, et al. Proof of principle of ocular sparing in dogs with sinonasal tumors treated with intensity-modulated radiation therapy. Vet Radiol Ultrasound 2010;51:561–70.
26. Castaldi P, Leccisotti L, Bussu F, et al. Role of (18)F-FDG PET-CT in head and neck squamous cell carcinoma. Acta Otorhinolaryngol Ital 2013;33:1–8.
27. Yoshikawa H, Randall EK, Kraft SL, et al. Comparison between 2-(18) F-Fluoro-2-Deoxy-D-glucose positron emission tomography and contrast-enhanced computed tomography for measuring gross tumor volume in cats with oral squamous cell carcinoma. Vet Radiol Ultrasound 2013;54:307–13.
28. Randall EK, Kraft SL, Yoshikawa H, et al. Evaluation of 18F-FDG PET/CT as a diagnostic imaging and staging tool for feline oral squamous cell carcinoma. Vet Comp Oncol 2013;54:307–13.
29. Hansen AE, Kristensen AT, Jorgensen JT, et al. (64)Cu-ATSM and (18)FDG PET uptake and (64)Cu-ATSM autoradiography in spontaneous canine tumors: comparison with pimonidazole hypoxia immunohistochemistry. Radiat Oncol 2012; 7:89.

30. Valdes-Martinez A, Kraft SL, Brundage CM, et al. Assessment of blood pool, soft tissue, and skeletal uptake of sodium fluoride F 18 with positron emission tomography-computed tomography in four clinically normal dogs. Am J Vet Res 2012;73:1589–95.
31. Nieset JR, Harmon JF, LaRue SM. Use of cone-beam computed tomography to characterize daily urinary bladder variations during fractionated radiotherapy for canine bladder cancer. Vet Radiol Ultrasound 2011;52:580–8.
32. Nolan MW, Kogan L, Griffin LR, et al. Intensity-modulated and image-guided radiation therapy for treatment of genitourinary carcinomas in dogs. J Vet Intern Med 2012;26:987–95.
33. Leksell L. The stereotaxic method and radiosurgery of the brain. Acta Chir Scand 1951;102:316–9.
34. Timmerman RD, Kavanagh BD, Cho LC, et al. Stereotactic body radiation therapy in multiple organ sites. J Clin Oncol 2007;25:947–52.
35. Timmerman RD, Bizekis CS, Pass HI, et al. Local surgical, ablative, and radiation treatment of metastases. CA Cancer J Clin 2009;59:145–70.
36. Lo SS, Fakiris AJ, Teh BS, et al. Stereotactic body radiation therapy for oligometastases. Expert Rev Anticancer Ther 2009;9:621–35.
37. Adler JR Jr, Chang SD, Murphy MJ, et al. The Cyberknife: a frameless robotic system for radiosurgery. Stereotact Funct Neurosurg 1997;69:124–8.
38. Farese JP, Milner R, Thompson MS, et al. Stereotactic radiosurgery for treatment of osteosarcomas involving the distal portions of the limbs in dogs. J Am Vet Med Assoc 2004;225:1567–72.
39. Ryan SD, Ehrhart NE, Worley D, et al. Stereotactic radiation therapy for appendicular bone tumors. Vet Radiol Ultrasound 2009;51(2):234.
40. Custis JT, Ryan SD, Valdes-Martinez A, et al. Identifying factors predictive of osteosarcoma related pathologic fracture following stereotactic radiation therapy. Vet Radiol Ultrasound 2009;51(2):234.
41. Custis JT, Harmon JF, Ryan SD, et al. Canine nasal tumors: a stereotactic radiation therapy approach. J Vet Intern Med 2011;25:746–47.
42. Griffin L, Custis JT, Nolan MW, et al. Stereotactic radiation therapy for intracalvarial tumors in dogs. Proceedings of the 2011 Veterinary Cancer Society. Albuquerque (NM): 2011. p. 116.
43. Lunn KF, LaRue SM. Endocrine function in cats after stereotactic radiosurgery treatment for acromegally. J Vet Intern Med 2009;23:698.

Immunotherapy in Veterinary Oncology

Philip J. Bergman, DVM, MS, PhD[a,b,*]

KEYWORDS

- Veterinary oncology • Tumor immunotherapy • Tumor immunology • DNA vaccine
- Xenogeneic DNA vaccine • Monoclonal antibody

KEY POINTS

- The immune system is generally divided into 2 primary components: the innate immune response and the highly specific, but more slowly developing, adaptive or acquired immune response.
- Immune responses can be further separated by whether they are induced by exposure to a foreign antigen (an active response) or are transferred through serum or lymphocytes from an immunized individual (a passive response).
- The ideal cancer immunotherapy agent should be able to discriminate between cancer and normal cells (ie, specificity), be potent enough to kill small or large numbers of tumor cells (ie, sensitivity), and, lastly, be able to prevent recurrence of the tumor (ie, durability).
- Tumor immunology and immunotherapy is one of the most exciting and rapidly expanding fields.

The term, *immunity*, is derived from the Latin word, *immunitas*, which refers to the legal protection afforded to Roman senators holding office. Although the immune system is normally thought of as providing protection against infectious disease (and much of this issue of *Veterinary Clinics of North America* is devoted to such), the immune system's ability to recognize and eliminate cancer is the fundamental rationale for the immunotherapy of cancer. Multiple lines of evidence support a role for the immune system in managing cancer, including (1) spontaneous remissions in cancer patients without treatment, (2) the presence of tumor-specific cytotoxic T cells within tumor or draining lymph nodes, (3) the presence of monocytic, lymphocytic, and plasmacytic cellular infiltrates in tumors, (4) the increased incidence of some types of cancer in immunosuppressed patients, and (5) documentation of cancer remissions with the use of immunomodulators.[1,2] With the tools of molecular biology and a greater understanding of mechanisms to harness the immune system, effective tumor

[a] Clinical Studies, VCA, 546 Bedford Road, Bedford Hills, New York, NY 10507, USA;
[b] Department of Molecular Pharmacology & Chemistry, Memorial Sloan-Kettering Cancer Center, 1275 York Avenue, New York, NY 10065, USA
* Memorial Sloan-Kettering Cancer Center, New York, NY.
E-mail address: philip.bergman@vcahospitals.com

Vet Clin Small Anim 44 (2014) 925–939
http://dx.doi.org/10.1016/j.cvsm.2014.05.002
0195-5616/14/$ – see front matter © 2014 Elsevier Inc. All rights reserved.

immunotherapy is becoming a reality. This new class of therapeutics offers a more targeted and, therefore, precise approach to the treatment of cancer. It is likely that immunotherapy will have a place alongside the classic cancer treatment triad components of surgery, radiation therapy, and chemotherapy within the next 5 to 10 years.

TUMOR IMMUNOLOGY
Cellular Components

The immune system is generally divided into 2 primary components: the innate immune response and the highly specific, but more slowly developing, adaptive or acquired immune response. Innate immunity is rapidly acting but typically not very specific and includes physicochemical barriers (eg, skin and mucosa); blood proteins, such as complement, phagocytic cells (macrophages, neutrophils, dendritic cells [DCs], and natural killer [NK] cells), and cytokines, which coordinate and regulate the cells involved in innate immunity. Adaptive immunity is thought of as the acquired arm of immunity, which allows for exquisite specificity, an ability to remember the previous existence of the pathogen (ie, memory) and differentiate self from nonself, and importantly the ability to respond more vigorously on repeat exposure to the pathogen. Adaptive immunity consists of T and B lymphocytes. The T cells are further divided into CD8 (cluster of differentiation) and major histocompatibility complex (MHC) class I cytotoxic helper T cells (CD4 and MHC class II), NK cells, and regulatory T cells. B lymphocytes produce antibodies (humoral system), which may activate complement, enhance phagocytosis of opsonized target cells, and induce antibody-dependent cellular cytotoxicity. B-cell responses to tumors are thought by many investigators to be less important than the development of T cell–mediated immunity, but there is little evidence to fully support this notion.[3] The innate and adaptive arms of immunity are not mutually exclusive; they are linked by (1) the innate response's ability to stimulate and influence the nature of the adaptive response and (2) the sharing of effector mechanisms between innate and adaptive immune responses.

Immune responses can be further separated by whether they are induced by exposure to a foreign antigen (an active response) or are transferred through serum or lymphocytes from an immunized individual (a passive response). Although both approaches have the ability to be extremely specific for an antigen of interest, one important difference is the inability of passive approaches to confer memory. The principal components of the active/adaptive immune system are lymphocytes, antigen-presenting cells, and effector cells. Furthermore, responses can be subdivided by whether they are specific for a certain antigen or a nonspecific response whereby immunity is attempted to be conferred by up-regulating the immune system without a specific target. These definitions are helpful because they allow methodologies to be more completely characterized, such as active-specific, passive-nonspecific, and so forth.

Immune Surveillance

The idea that the immune system may actively prevent the development of neoplasia is termed, *cancer immunosurveillance*. Sound scientific evidence supports some aspects of this hypothesis,[4–7] including (1) interferon (IFN)-γ protecting mice against the growth of tumors, (2) mice lacking IFN-γ receptor are more sensitive to chemically induced sarcomas than normal mice and more likely to spontaneously develop tumors, (3) mice lacking major components of the adaptive immune response (T and B cells) having a high rate of spontaneous tumors, and (4) mice lacking IFN-γ and B/T cells developing tumors, especially at a young age.

Immune Evasion by Tumors

There are significant barriers to the generation of effective antitumor immunity by the host. Many tumors evade surveillance mechanisms and grow in immunocompetent hosts, easily illustrated by the overwhelming numbers of people and animals succumbing to cancer. There are multiple ways in which tumors evade the immune response, including (1) immunosuppressive cytokine production (eg, transforming growth factor [TGF]-β and interleukin [IL]-10)[8,9]; (2) impaired DC function via inactivation (anergy) and/or poor DC maturation through changes in IL-6/IL-10/vascular endothelial growth factor/granulocyte-macrophage colony-stimulating factor[10]; (3) induction of cells called regulatory T cells, which were initially called suppressor T cells (CD4/CD25/CTLA-4/GITR/Foxp3–positive cells, which can suppress tumor-specific CD4/CD8$^+$ T cells)[11]; (4) MHC I loss through structural defects, changes in β$_2$-microglobulin synthesis, defects in transporter-associated antigen processing, or actual MHC I gene loss (ie, allelic or locus loss); and (5) MHC I antigen presentation loss through B7-1 attenuation (B7-1 is an important costimulatory molecule for CD28-mediated T-cell receptor and MHC engagement) when the MHC system in #4 remains intact.

NONSPECIFIC TUMOR IMMUNOTHERAPY

Dr William Coley, a New York surgeon in the early 1900s, noted that some cancer patients developing incidental bacterial infections survived longer than those without infection.[12] Coley developed a bacterial "toxin" (killed cultures of Serratia marcescens and Streptococcus pyogenes: Coley's toxins) to treat people with sarcomas, which provided complete response rates of approximately 15%. Unfortunately, high failure rates and significant side effects led to discontinuation of this approach. His seminal work laid the foundation for nonspecific modulation of the immune response in the treatment of cancer. There are numerous nonspecific tumor immunotherapy approaches ranging from biologic response modifiers (BRMs) to recombinant cytokines (discussed later).

Biologic Response Modifiers

BRMs are molecules that can modify the biologic response of cells to changes in its external environment, which in the context of cancer immunotherapy could easily span nonspecific and specific immunotherapies. This section discusses nonspecific BRMs (sometimes termed, *immunopotentiators*), which are often related to bacteria and/or viruses.

One of the earliest BRM discoveries after Coley's toxin was the use of bacille Calmette-Guérin (BCG); interestingly, Guérin was a veterinarian. BCG is the live attenuated strain of *Mycobacterium bovis*, and intravesical instillation in the urinary bladder causes a significant local inflammatory response, which results in antitumor responses.[13] The use of BCG in veterinary patients was first reported by Owen and Bostock[14] in 1974 and has been investigated with many types of cancers, including urinary bladder carcinoma, osteosarcoma, lymphoma, prostatic carcinoma, transmissible venereal tumor, mammary tumors, sarcoids, squamous cell carcinoma, and others.[15–18] LDI-100, a product containing BCG and human chorionic gonadotropin, was compared with vinblastine in dogs with measurable grade II or III mast cell tumors.[19] Response rates were 28.6% and 11.7%, respectively, and the LDI-100 group had significantly less neutropenia. It is exciting for the field of veterinary cancer immunotherapy to potentially be able to use a BRM product that has greater efficacy and less toxicity than a chemotherapy standard of care. Unfortunately, LDI-100 is not commercially available at present.

Corynebacterium parvum is another BRM that has been investigated for several tumors in veterinary medicine, including melanoma and mammary carcinoma.[20,21] Other bacterially derived BRMs include attenuated *Salmonella typhimurium* (VNP20009), mycobacterial cell wall DNA complexes (abstracts only at present), and bacterial superantigens.[22,23] Mycobacterial cell walls contain muramyl dipeptide (MDP), which can activate monocytes and tissue macrophages. Muramyl tripeptide phosphatidylethanolamine (MTP-PE) is an analog of MDP. When encapsulated in multilamellar liposomes (L-MTP-PE), monocytes and macrophages uptake muramyl tripeptide, leading to activation and subsequent tumoricidal effects through induction of multiple cytokines, including IL-1a, IL-1b, IL-7, IL-8, IL-12, and tumor necrosis factor.[24] L-MTP-PE has been investigated in many tumors in human and veterinary patients, including osteosarcoma, hemangiosarcoma, and mammary carcinoma.[24–28]

Oncolytic viruses have also been used as nonspecific anticancer BRMs in human and veterinary patients.[29] Adenoviruses have been engineered to transcriptionally target canine osteosarcoma cells and have been tested in vitro and in normal dogs with no major signs of virus-associated side effects.[30–32] Similarly, canine distemper virus (CDV), the canine equivalent of human measles virus, has been used in vitro to infect canine lymphocyte cell lines and neoplastic lymphocytes from dogs with B- and T-cell lymphoma,[33] with high infectivity rates, suggesting that CDV may be investigated in the future for treatment of dogs with lymphoma.

Imiquimod (Aldara) is a novel BRM that is a Toll-like receptor 7 agonist.[34] Imiquimod has been reported as a successful treatment of Bowen disease (multicentric squamous cell carcinoma in situ) and other skin diseases in humans. Twelve cats with Bowen-like disease were treated topically with imiquimod 5% cream and initial as well as all subsequent new lesions responded in all cats.[35] An additional cat (with pinnal actinic keratoses and squamous cell carcinoma) and dog with cutaneous melanocytomas have subsequently been reported to have been successfully treated with topical imiquimod 5% cream.[36,37] It seems, therefore, that imiquimod 5% cream is well tolerated, and further studies are warranted to further examine its usefulness in cats and dogs with other skin tumors that are not treatable through standardized means.

Recombinant Cytokines, Growth Factors, and Hormones

Several investigations using recombinant cytokines, growth factors, or hormones in various fashions for human and veterinary cancer patients have been reported to date. Many have investigated the in vitro and/or in vivo effects of the soluble cytokine (eg, interferons, IL-2, IL-12, and IL-15)[38–49] or liposome encapsulation of the cytokine (eg, liposomal IL-2)[39,50–53] or use a virus, cell, liposome-DNA complex, plasmid, or other mechanism to expresses the cytokine (eg, recombinant poxvirus expressing IL-2).[50,54–61] The European Committee for Medicinal Products for Veterinary Use adopted a positive opinion in March 2013 for the veterinary product, Oncept IL-2 (feline poxvirus expressing recombinant feline IL-2). It is to be used in addition to surgery and radiation in cats with large fibrosarcomas without metastasis or lymph node involvement, to reduce the risk of relapse and increase the time to relapse.

CANCER VACCINES

The ultimate goal for a cancer vaccine is elicitation of an antitumor immune response that results in clinical regression of a tumor and/or its metastases. There are many types of tumor vaccines in phase I–III trials across a wide range of tumor types. Responses to cancer vaccines may take several months or more to appear due to the slower speed of induction of the adaptive arm of the immune system (outlined in **Table 1**).

Treatment Type	Mechanism of Action	Specificity	Sensitivity	Response Time	Durability of Response
Chemotherapy	Cytotoxicity	Poor	Variable	Hours–days	Variable
Antitumor vaccine	Immune response	Good	Good	Weeks–months	Variable–long

Table 1
Comparison of chemotherapy and antitumor vaccines

The immune system detects tumors through specific tumor-associated antigens (TAAs) and/or abnormal disease-associated antigens (DAAs) that are potentially recognized by both CTLs and antibodies.[62,63] TAAs and/or DAAs may be common to a particular tumor type; be unique to an individual tumor; or may arise from mutated gene products, such as ras, p53, p21, and others. Although unique TAAs may be more immunogenic than the other aforementioned shared tumor antigens, they are not practical targets because of their narrow specificity. Most shared tumor antigens are normal cellular antigens that are overexpressed in tumors. The first group to be identified was termed, *cancer testes antigens*, due to expression in normal testes, but they are also found in melanoma and various other solid tumors, such as the MAGE/BAGE gene family. This article highlights those tumor vaccine approaches that seem to hold particular promise in human clinical trials and many that have been tested to date in veterinary medicine.

A variety of approaches have been taken to date to focus the immune system on the aforementioned targets, including (1) whole-cell, tumor cell lysate, and/or subunit vaccines (autologous, or made from a patient's own tumor tissue; allogeneic, or made from individuals within a species bearing the same type of cancer; or whole-cell vaccines from γ-irradiated tumor cell lines with or without immunostimulatory cytokines),[56,64–74] (2) DNA vaccines that immunize with syngeneic and/or xenogeneic (different species from recipient) plasmid DNA designed to elicit antigen-specific humoral and cellular immunity[75–77] (discussed later), (3) viral vector-based methodologies designed to deliver genes encoding TAAs and/or immunostimulatory cytokines,[78–82] (4) DC or CD40-activated B-cell vaccines (which are commonly loaded or transfected with TAAs, DNA or RNA from TAAs, or tumor lysates),[83–90] (5) adoptive cell transfer (the "transfer" of specific populations of immune effector cells to generate a more powerful and focused antitumor immune response), and (6) antibody approaches, such as monoclonal antibodies,[91] anti-idiotype antibodies (an idiotype is an immunoglobulin sequence unique to each B lymphocyte, and therefore antibodies directed against these idiotypes are referred to as anti-idiotype), or conjugated antibodies. The ideal cancer immunotherapy agent would be able to discriminate between cancer and normal cells (ie specificity), be potent enough to kill small or large numbers of tumor cells (ie sensitivity), and, lastly, be able to prevent recurrence of the tumor (ie durability).

This author has developed a xenogeneic DNA vaccine program for melanoma in collaboration with human investigators from Memorial Sloan Kettering Cancer Center.[92,93] Preclinical and clinical studies by the author's laboratory and others have shown that xenogeneic DNA vaccination with tyrosinase family members (eg, tyrosinase, GP100, and GP75) can produce immune responses resulting in tumor rejection or protection and prolongation of survival whereas syngeneic vaccination with orthologous DNA does not induce immune responses. Although tyrosinase may not seem to be a preferred target in amelanotic canine melanoma due to poor expression when assessed by immunohistochemistry (IHC),[94] more appropriate/sensitive PCR-based studies and other IHC-based studies document significant tyrosinase overexpression in melanotic and amelanotic melanomas across species.[95–100] These studies provided the impetus for development of a xenogeneic tyrosinase (or similar melanosomal glycoproteins) DNA vaccine program in canine malignant melanoma (CMM). Cohorts of dogs received increasing doses of xenogeneic plasmid DNA encoding either human tyrosinase (huTyr), murine GP75, murine tyrosinase (muTyr), muTyr ± human granulocyte-monocyte (HuGM)-CSF (both administered as plasmid DNA), or muTyr off-study intramuscularly biweekly for a total of 4 vaccinations. The author and collaborators have investigated the antibody and T-cell responses in dogs vaccinated with huTyr. Antigen-specific (huTyr) IFN-γ T cells were found along with 2- to 5-fold increases in circulating antibodies to huTyr, which can cross-react to canine tyrosinase, suggesting the breaking of tolerance.[101,102] The clinical results with prolongation in survival have been reported previously.[92,93] The results of these trials demonstrate that xenogeneic DNA vaccination in CMM (1) is safe, (2) leads to the development of anti-tyrosinase antibodies and T cells, (3) is potentially therapeutic, and (4) is an attractive candidate for further evaluation in an adjuvant, minimal residual disease phase II setting for CMM. Based on these studies, a multi-institutional safety and efficacy trial for US Department of Agriculture (USDA) licensure in dogs with locally controlled stage II/III oral melanoma was initiated in 2006 with granting of conditional licensure in 2007, which represented the first US governmental regulatory agency approval of a vaccine to treat cancer across species. Results of this licensure trial documented a statistically significant improvement in survival for vaccinates versus controls and a full licensure for the HuTyr-based canine melanoma vaccine from the USDA Center for Veterinary Biologics was received in December 2009 (Oncept, Merial, Duluth, GA).[103]

Kaser-Hotz and colleagues[104] reported on concurrent use of Oncept and external beam radiation because many dogs with oral malignant melanoma may not be able to undergo surgery for local tumor control. This pilot study determined that concurrent use was well tolerated with no unexpected toxicities. Ottnod and colleagues[105] performed a single-site retrospective study on 30 dogs with stage II to III oral malignant melanoma (15 each with and without use of Oncept). They determined that those dogs receiving Oncept did not achieve a greater progression-free survival, disease-free interval, or median survival time than dogs that did not receive the vaccine. Contrary to the aforementioned prospective USDA 5-site licensure trial,[103] this study had less than 35% of cases treated surgically with margins 1 mm or more, suggesting a significant lack of local tumor control. Furthermore, contrary to the aforementioned prospective USDA 5-site licensure trial, the Ottnod and colleagues study, similar to most noncontrolled retrospective studies, had a wide variety of other treatments used in both the nonvaccinated and vaccinated groups and the cause (in the context of local or distant disease) of death and/or progression of disease was not reported.

Human clinical trials using various xenogeneic melanosomal antigens as DNA (or peptide with adjuvant) vaccination began in 2005 and the preliminary results look favorable.[106–108] To further highlight xenogeneic DNA vaccination as a platform to target other possible antigens for other histologies, the authors and colleagues have completed a phase I trial of murine CD20 for dogs with B-cell lymphoma; will be initiating additional trials, such as a phase I trial of rat HER2 and a phase II trial of murine CD20; and have also investigated the efficacy of local tumor control and use of xenogeneic DNA vaccination in dogs with digit malignant melanoma.[109] These investigations led to the development of a canine digit melanoma staging scheme and found an improvement in survival compared with historical outcomes with digit amputation only. The authors and colleagues also documented a decreased prognosis for dogs with advanced stage disease and/or increased time from digit amputation to the start of vaccination. Phillips and co-investigators[95,110] have also recently reported the over-expression of tyrosinase in equine melanoma, determined the safety and optimal use of the needle-free delivery device into the pectoral region with Oncept, and documented antigen-specific humoral responses after vaccination in all horses.

Tumor immunology and immunotherapy is one of the most exciting and rapidly expanding fields at present. Significant resources are focused on mechanisms to simultaneously maximally stimulate an antitumor immune response while minimizing the immunosuppressive aspects of the tumor microenvironment.[8] The recent elucidation and blockade of immunosuppressive cytokines (eg, TGF-β, IL-10, and IL-13) and/or the negative costimulatory molecule CTLA-4[111,112] along with the functional characterization of myeloid-derived suppressor cells and regulatory T cells[113–116] may dramatically improve cell-mediated immunity to tumors. As investigators more easily generate specific antitumor immune responses in patients, they need to remain vigilant to not push the immune system into pathologic autoimmunity. In addition, immunotherapy is unlikely to become a sole modality in the treatment of cancer because the traditional modalities of surgery, radiation, and/or chemotherapy are likely to be used in combination with immunotherapy in the future. Like any form of anticancer treatment, immunotherapy seems to work best in a minimal residual disease setting, suggesting its most appropriate use will be in an adjuvant setting with local tumor therapies, such as surgery and/or radiation.[117] Similarly, the long-held belief that chemotherapy (noncorticosteroid) attenuates immune responses from cancer vaccines is beginning to be disproved through investigations on a variety of levels.[118,119]

Additional exciting new approaches that seem to confer a survival benefit in human metastatic melanoma include the use of the anti–CTLA-4 antibody, ipilimumab (Yervoy, Bristol-Myers Squibb, New Jersey, USA), and the selective BRAF inhibitors, vemurafenib (Zelboraf, Genetech, California, USA) and dabrafenib (GSK2118436, GlaxoSmithKline, North Carolina, USA), in patients who are BRAF V600 mutation positive; 53% of human patients receiving concurrent administration of ipilimumab and a new antibody directed against human programmed cell death 1 receptor, nivolumab, had an objective tumor response with tumor reductions of 80% or greater.[120] Because a small subset of dogs with malignant melanoma has exon 11 KIT gene mutations,[121,122] the more routine use of KIT testing by polymerase chain reaction (PCR) of CMM and subsequent use of c-kit small molecule inhibitors (particularly in dogs with advanced-stage disease and/or lack of response to Oncept) should be considered. Furthermore, with somatic mutations in NRAS and PTEN found in canine malignant melanoma[123] similar to human melanoma hotspot sites, these may represent logical druggable targets in the future.

In summary, the future looks bright for immunotherapy. The veterinary oncology profession is uniquely able to greatly contribute to the many advances to come in this field. Unfortunately, what works in a mouse often does not reflect the outcome in human cancer patients. Therefore, comparative immunotherapy studies using veterinary patients may be able to better bridge murine and human studies. To this end, many cancers in dogs and cats seem remarkably stronger models for counterpart human tumors than currently available murine model systems.[123–127] This is likely due to a variety of reasons, including, but not limited to, extreme similarities in the biology of the tumors (chemoresistance, radioresistance, sharing metastatic phenotypes and site selectivity, and so forth), spontaneous syngeneic cancer (vs typically an induced and/or xenogeneic cancer in murine models), and finally that the dogs and cats that are spontaneously developing these tumors are outbred, immune competent, and live in the same environment as humans. This author ardently looks forward to the time when immunotherapy plays a significant role in the treatment and/ or prevention of cancer in human and veterinary patients.

REFERENCES

1. Bergman PJ. Biologic response modification. In: Rosenthal RC, editor. Veterinary oncology secrets. 1st edition. Philadelphia: Hanley & Belfus, Inc; 2001. p. 79–82.
2. Baxevanis CN, Perez SA, Papamichail M. Cancer immunotherapy. Crit Rev Clin Lab Sci 2009;46:167–89.
3. Reilly RT, Emens LA, Jaffee EM. Humoral and cellular immune responses: independent forces or collaborators in the fight against cancer? Curr Opin Investig Drugs 2001;2(1):133–5.
4. Smyth MJ, Godfrey DI, Trapani JA. A fresh look at tumor immunosurveillance and immunotherapy. Nat Immunol 2001;2(4):293–9.
5. Wallace ME, Smyth MJ. The role of natural killer cells in tumor control–effectors and regulators of adaptive immunity. Springer Semin Immunopathol 2005;27(1): 49–64.
6. Itoh H, Horiuchi Y, Nagasaki T, et al. Evaluation of immunological status in tumor-bearing dogs. Vet Immunol Immunopathol 2009;132(2–4):85–90.
7. Schmiedt CW, Grimes JA, Holzman G, et al. Incidence and risk factors for development of malignant neoplasia after feline renal transplantation and cyclosporine-based immunosuppression. Vet Comp Oncol 2009;7:45–53.
8. Catchpole B, Gould SM, Kellett-Gregory LM, et al. Immunosuppressive cytokines in the regional lymph node of a dog suffering from oral malignant melanoma. J Small Anim Pract 2002;43(10):464–7.
9. Zagury D, Gallo RC. Anti-cytokine Ab immune therapy: present status and perspectives. Drug Discov Today 2004;9(2):72–81.
10. Morse MA, Mosca PJ, Clay TM, et al. Dendritic cell maturation in active immunotherapy strategies. Expert Opin Biol Ther 2002;2(1):35–43.
11. Yamaguchi T, Sakaguchi S. Regulatory T cells in immune surveillance and treatment of cancer. Semin Cancer Biol 2006;16(2):115–23.
12. Richardson MA, Ramirez T, Russell NC, et al. Coley toxins immunotherapy: a retrospective review. Altern Ther Health Med 1999;5(3):42–7.
13. Herr HW, Morales A. History of bacillus Calmette-Guerin and bladder cancer: an immunotherapy success story. J Urol 2008;179:53–6.
14. Owen LN, Bostock DE. Proceedings: tumour therapy in dogs using B.C.G. Br J Cancer 1974;29:95.
15. MacEwen EG. An immunologic approach to the treatment of cancer. Vet Clin North Am 1977;7:65–75.
16. Theilen GH, Hills D. Comparative aspects of cancer immunotherapy: immunologic methods used for treatment of spontaneous cancer in animals. J Am Vet Med Assoc 1982;181:1134–41.
17. MacEwen EG. Approaches to cancer therapy using biological response modifiers. Vet Clin North Am Small Anim Pract 1985;15:667–88.
18. Klein WR, Rutten VP, Steerenberg PA, et al. The present status of BCG treatment in the veterinary practice. In Vivo 1991;5:605–8.
19. Henry CJ, Downing S, Rosenthal RC, et al. Evaluation of a novel immunomodulator composed of human chorionic gonadotropin and bacillus Calmette-Guerin for treatment of canine mast cell tumors in clinically affected dogs. Am J Vet Res 2007;68:1246–51.

20. Parodi AL, Misdorp W, Mialot JP, et al. Intratumoral BCG and Corynebacterium parvum therapy of canine mammary tumours before radical mastectomy. Cancer Immunol Immunother 1983;15:172–7.
21. MacEwen EG, Patnaik AK, Harvey HJ, et al. Canine oral melanoma: comparison of surgery versus surgery plus corynebacterium parvum. Cancer Invest 1986; 4(5):397–402.
22. Thamm DH, Kurzman ID, King I, et al. Systemic administration of an attenuated, tumor-targeting Salmonella typhimurium to dogs with spontaneous neoplasia: phase I evaluation. Clin Cancer Res 2005;11:4827–34.
23. Dow SW, Elmslie RE, Willson AP, et al. In vivo tumor transfection with superantigen plus cytokine genes induces tumor regression and prolongs survival in dogs with malignant melanoma. J Clin Invest 1998;101:2406–14.
24. Kleinerman ES, Jia SF, Griffin J, et al. Phase II study of liposomal muramyl tripeptide in osteosarcoma: the cytokine cascade and monocyte activation following administration. J Clin Oncol 1992;10:1310–6.
25. MacEwen EG, Kurzman ID, Vail DM, et al. Adjuvant therapy for melanoma in dogs: results of randomized clinical trials using surgery, liposome-encapsulated muramyl tripeptide, and granulocyte macrophage colony-stimulating factor. Clin Cancer Res 1999;5:4249–58.
26. Teske E, Rutteman GR, vd Ingh TS, et al. Liposome-encapsulated muramyl tripeptide phosphatidylethanolamine (L-MTP-PE): a randomized clinical trial in dogs with mammary carcinoma. Anticancer Res 1998;18:1015–9.
27. Kurzman ID, MacEwen EG, Rosenthal RC, et al. Adjuvant therapy for osteosarcoma in dogs: results of randomized clinical trials using combined liposome-encapsulated muramyl tripeptide and cisplatin. Clin Cancer Res 1995;1: 1595–601.
28. Vail DM, MacEwen EG, Kurzman ID, et al. Liposome-encapsulated muramyl tripeptide phosphatidylethanolamine adjuvant immunotherapy for splenic hemangiosarcoma in the dog: a randomized multi-institutional clinical trial. Clin Cancer Res 1995;1:1165–70.
29. Arendt M, Nasir L, Morgan IM. Oncolytic gene therapy for canine cancers: teaching old dog viruses new tricks. Vet Comp Oncol 2009;7:153–61.
30. Smith BF, Curiel DT, Ternovoi VV, et al. Administration of a conditionally replicative oncolytic canine adenovirus in normal dogs. Cancer Biother Radiopharm 2006;21:601–6.
31. Le LP, Rivera AA, Glasgow JN, et al. Infectivity enhancement for adenoviral transduction of canine osteosarcoma cells. Gene Ther 2006;13:389–99.
32. Hemminki A, Kanerva A, Kremer EJ, et al. A canine conditionally replicating adenovirus for evaluating oncolytic virotherapy in a syngeneic animal model. Mol Ther 2003;7:163–73.
33. Suter SE, Chein MB, von M, et al. In vitro canine distemper virus infection of canine lymphoid cells: a prelude to oncolytic therapy for lymphoma. Clin Cancer Res 2005;11:1579–87.
34. Meyer T, Stockfleth E. Clinical investigations of Toll-like receptor agonists. Expert Opin Investig Drugs 2008;17:1051–65.
35. Gill VL, Bergman PJ, Baer KE, et al. Use of imiquimod 5% cream (AldaraTM) in cats with multicentric squamous cell carcinoma in situ: 12 cases (2002-2005). Vet Comp Oncol 2008;6:55–64.
36. Peters-Kennedy J, Scott DW, Miller WH Jr. Apparent clinical resolution of pinnal actinic keratoses and squamous cell carcinoma in a cat using topical imiquimod 5% cream. J Feline Med Surg 2008;10(6):593–9.

37. Coyner K, Loeffler D. Topical imiquimod in the treatment of two cutaneous melanocytomas in a dog. Vet Dermatol 2012;23(2):145–9 e31.
38. Tateyama S, Priosoeryanto BP, Yamaguchi R, et al. In vitro growth inhibition activities of recombinant feline interferon on all lines derived from canine tumors. Res Vet Sci 1995;59:275–7.
39. Kruth SA. Biological response modifiers: interferons, interleukins, recombinant products, liposomal products. Vet Clin North Am Small Anim Pract 1998;28: 269–95.
40. Whitley EM, Bird AC, Zucker KE, et al. Modulation by canine interferon-gamma of major histocompatibility complex and tumor-associated antigen expression in canine mammary tumor and melanoma cell lines. Anticancer Res 1995;15: 923–9.
41. Hampel V, Schwarz B, Kempf C, et al. Adjuvant immunotherapy of feline fibrosarcoma with recombinant feline interferon-omega. J Vet Intern Med 2007;21: 1340–6.
42. Finocchiaro LM, Glikin GC. Cytokine-enhanced vaccine and suicide gene therapy as surgery adjuvant treatments for spontaneous canine melanoma. Gene Ther 2008;15:267–76.
43. Cutrera J, Torrero M, Shiomitsu K, et al. Intratumoral bleomycin and IL-12 electrochemogenetherapy for treating head and neck tumors in dogs. Methods Mol Biol 2008;423:319–25.
44. Finocchiaro LM, Fiszman GL, Karara AL, et al. Suicide gene and cytokines combined nonviral gene therapy for spontaneous canine melanoma. Cancer Gene Ther 2008;15:165–72.
45. Akhtar N, Padilla ML, Dickerson EB, et al. Interleukin-12 inhibits tumor growth in a novel angiogenesis canine hemangiosarcoma xenograft model. Neoplasia 2004;6:106–16.
46. Dickerson EB, Fosmire S, Padilla ML, et al. Potential to target dysregulated interleukin-2 receptor expression in canine lymphoid and hematopoietic malignancies as a model for human cancer. J Immunother 2002;25:36–45.
47. Okano F, Yamada K. Canine interleukin-18 induces apoptosis and enhances Fas ligand mRNA expression in a canine carcinoma cell line. Anticancer Res 2000; 20:3411–5.
48. Jahnke A, Hirschberger J, Fischer C, et al. Intra-tumoral gene delivery of feIL-2, feIFN-gamma and feGM-CSF using magnetofection as a neoadjuvant treatment option for feline fibrosarcomas: a phase-I study. J Vet Med A Physiol Pathol Clin Med 2007;54:599–606.
49. Dickerson EB, Akhtar N, Steinberg H, et al. Enhancement of the antiangiogenic activity of interleukin-12 by peptide targeted delivery of the cytokine to alphav-beta3 integrin. Mol Cancer Res 2004;2:663–73.
50. Dow S, Elmslie R, Kurzman I, et al. Phase I study of liposome-DNA complexes encoding the interleukin-2 gene in dogs with osteosarcoma lung metastases. Hum Gene Ther 2005;16:937–46.
51. Skubitz KM, Anderson PM. Inhalational interleukin-2 liposomes for pulmonary metastases: a phase I clinical trial. Anticancer Drugs 2000;11:555–63.
52. Khanna C, Anderson PM, Hasz DE, et al. Interleukin-2 liposome inhalation therapy is safe and effective for dogs with spontaneous pulmonary metastases. Cancer 1997;79:1409–21.
53. Khanna C, Hasz DE, Klausner JS, et al. Aerosol delivery of interleukin 2 liposomes is nontoxic and biologically effective: canine studies. Clin Cancer Res 1996;2:721–34.

54. Jourdier TM, Moste C, Bonnet MC, et al. Local immunotherapy of spontaneous feline fibrosarcomas using recombinant poxviruses expressing interleukin 2 (IL2). Gene Ther 2003;10(26):2126–32.
55. Siddiqui F, Li CY, Zhang X, et al. Characterization of a recombinant adenovirus vector encoding heat-inducible feline interleukin-12 for use in hyperthermia-induced gene-therapy. Int J Hyperthermia 2006;22:117–34.
56. Quintin-Colonna F, Devauchelle P, Fradelizi D, et al. Gene therapy of spontaneous canine melanoma and feline fibrosarcoma by intratumoral administration of histoincompatible cells expressing human interleukin-2. Gene Ther 1996; 3(12):1104–12.
57. Kamstock D, Guth A, Elmslie R, et al. Liposome-DNA complexes infused intravenously inhibit tumor angiogenesis and elicit antitumor activity in dogs with soft tissue sarcoma. Cancer Gene Ther 2006;13:306–17.
58. Junco JA, Basalto R, Fuentes F, et al. Gonadotrophin releasing hormone-based vaccine, an effective candidate for prostate cancer and other hormone-sensitive neoplasms. Adv Exp Med Biol 2008;617:581–7.
59. Chou PC, Chuang TF, Jan TR, et al. Effects of immunotherapy of IL-6 and IL-15 plasmids on transmissible venereal tumor in beagles. Vet Immunol Immunopathol 2009;130(1–2):25–34.
60. Chuang TF, Lee SC, Liao KW, et al. Electroporation-mediated IL-12 gene therapy in a transplantable canine cancer model. Int J Cancer 2009;125(3):698–707.
61. Finocchiaro LM, Glikin GC. Cytokine-enhanced vaccine and suicide gene therapy as surgery adjuvant treatments for spontaneous canine melanoma: 9 years of follow-up. Cancer Gene Ther 2012;19(12):852–61.
62. Bergman PJ. Anticancer vaccines. Vet Clin North Am Small Anim Pract 2007;37: 1111–9.
63. Beatty PL, Finn OJ. Preventing cancer by targeting abnormally expressed self-antigens: MUC1 vaccines for prevention of epithelial adenocarcinomas. Ann N Y Acad Sci 2013;1284:52–6.
64. Hogge GS, Burkholder JK, Culp J, et al. Preclinical development of human granulocyte-macrophage colony-stimulating factor-transfected melanoma cell vaccine using established canine cell lines and normal dogs. Cancer Gene Ther 1999;6(1):26–36.
65. Alexander AN, Huelsmeyer MK, Mitzey A, et al. Development of an allogeneic whole-cell tumor vaccine expressing xenogeneic gp100 and its implementation in a phase II clinical trial in canine patients with malignant melanoma. Cancer Immunol Immunother 2006;55(4):433–42.
66. U'Ren LW, Biller BJ, Elmslie RE, et al. Evaluation of a novel tumor vaccine in dogs with hemangiosarcoma. J Vet Intern Med 2007;21:113–20.
67. Bird RC, Deinnocentes P, Lenz S, et al. An allogeneic hybrid-cell fusion vaccine against canine mammary cancer. Vet Immunol Immunopathol 2008;123:289–304.
68. Turek MM, Thamm DH, Mitzey A, et al. Human granulocyte & macrophage colony-stimulating factor DNA cationic-lipid complexed autologous tumour cell vaccination in the treatment of canine B-cell multicentric lymphoma. Vet Comp Oncol 2007;5:219–31.
69. Kuntsi-Vaattovaara H, Verstraete FJ, Newsome JT, et al. Resolution of persistent oral papillomatosis in a dog after treatment with a recombinant canine oral papillomavirus vaccine. Vet Comp Oncol 2003;1:57–63.
70. Milner RJ, Salute M, Crawford C, et al. The immune response to disialoganglioside GD3 vaccination in normal dogs: a melanoma surface antigen vaccine. Vet Immunol Immunopathol 2006;114:273–84.

71. Marconato L, Frayssinet P, Rouquet N, et al. Randomized, placebo-controlled, double-blinded chemo-immunotherapy clinical trial in a Pet Dog model of Diffuse Large B-cell Lymphoma. Clin Cancer Res 2013;20(3):668–77.

72. Suckow MA. Cancer vaccines: harnessing the potential of anti-tumor immunity. Vet J 2013;198(1):28–33.

73. Epple LM, Bemis LT, Cavanaugh RP, et al. Prolonged remission of advanced bronchoalveolar adenocarcinoma in a dog treated with autologous, tumour-derived chaperone-rich cell lysate (CRCL) vaccine. Int J Hyperthermia 2013; 29(5):390–8.

74. Andersen BM, Pluhar GE, Seiler CE, et al. Vaccination for invasive canine meningioma induces in situ production of antibodies capable of antibody-dependent cell-mediated cytotoxicity. Cancer Res 2013;73(10):2987–97.

75. Kamstock D, Elmslie R, Thamm D, et al. Evaluation of a xenogeneic VEGF vaccine in dogs with soft tissue sarcoma. Cancer Immunol Immunother 2007;56: 1299–309.

76. Yu WY, Chuang TF, Guichard C, et al. Chicken HSP70 DNA vaccine inhibits tumor growth in a canine cancer model. Vaccine 2011;29(18):3489–500.

77. Impellizeri JA, Ciliberto G, Aurisicchio L. Electro-gene-transfer as a new tool for cancer immunotherapy in animals. Vet Comp Oncol 2012. [Epub ahead of print].

78. von EH, Sadeghi A, Carlsson B, et al. Efficient adenovector CD40 ligand immunotherapy of canine malignant melanoma. J Immunother 2008;31:377–84.

79. Johnston KB, Monteiro JM, Schultz LD, et al. Protection of beagle dogs from mucosal challenge with canine oral papillomavirus by immunization with recombinant adenoviruses expressing codon-optimized early genes. Virology 2005; 336:208–18.

80. Thacker EE, Nakayama M, Smith BF, et al. A genetically engineered adenovirus vector targeted to CD40 mediates transduction of canine dendritic cells and promotes antigen-specific immune responses in vivo. Vaccine 2009;27(50): 7116–24.

81. Peruzzi D, Mesiti G, Ciliberto G, et al. Telomerase and HER-2/neu as targets of genetic cancer vaccines in dogs. Vaccine 2010;28(5):1201–8.

82. Gavazza A, Lubas G, Fridman A, et al. Safety and efficacy of a genetic vaccine targeting telomerase plus chemotherapy for the therapy of canine B-cell lymphoma. Hum Gene Ther 2013;24(8):728–38.

83. Gyorffy S, Rodriguez-Lecompte JC, Woods JP, et al. Bone marrow-derived dendritic cell vaccination of dogs with naturally occurring melanoma by using human gp100 antigen. J Vet Intern Med 2005;19(1):56–63.

84. Tamura K, Arai H, Ueno E, et al. Comparison of dendritic cell-mediated immune responses among canine malignant cells. J Vet Med Sci 2007;69:925–30.

85. Tamura K, Yamada M, Isotani M, et al. Induction of dendritic cell-mediated immune responses against canine malignant melanoma cells. Vet J 2008;175: 126–9.

86. Rodriguez-Lecompte JC, Kruth S, Gyorffy S, et al. Cell-based cancer gene therapy: breaking tolerance or inducing autoimmunity? Anim Health Res Rev 2004; 5:227–34.

87. Kyte JA, Mu L, Aamdal S, et al. Phase I/II trial of melanoma therapy with dendritic cells transfected with autologous tumor-mRNA. Cancer Gene Ther 2006; 13:905–18.

88. Mason NJ, Coughlin CM, Overley B, et al. RNA-loaded CD40-activated B cells stimulate antigen-specific T-cell responses in dogs with spontaneous lymphoma. Gene Ther 2008;15:955–65.

89. Sorenmo KU, Krick E, Coughlin CM, et al. CD40-activated B cell cancer vaccine improves second clinical remission and survival in privately owned dogs with non-Hodgkin's lymphoma. PLoS One 2011;6(8):e24167.

90. Bird RC, Deinnocentes P, Church Bird AE, et al. An autologous dendritic cell canine mammary tumor hybrid-cell fusion vaccine. Cancer Immunol Immunother 2011;60(1):87–97.

91. Jeglum KA. Chemoimmunotherapy of canine lymphoma with adjuvant canine monoclonal antibody 231. Vet Clin North Am Small Anim Pract 1996;26(1):73–85.

92. Bergman PJ, Camps-Palau MA, McKnight JA, et al. Development of a xenogeneic DNA vaccine program for canine malignant melanoma at the Animal Medical Center. Vaccine 2006;24(21):4582–5.

93. Bergman PJ, McKnight J, Novosad A, et al. Long-term survival of dogs with advanced malignant melanoma after DNA vaccination with xenogeneic human tyrosinase: a phase I trial. Clin Cancer Res 2003;9(4):1284–90.

94. Smedley RC, Lamoureux J, Sledge DG, et al. Immunohistochemical diagnosis of canine oral amelanotic melanocytic neoplasms. Vet Pathol 2011;48(1):32–40.

95. Phillips JC, Lembcke LM, Noltenius CE, et al. Evaluation of tyrosinase expression in canine and equine melanocytic tumors. Am J Vet Res 2012;73(2):272–8.

96. Cangul IT, van Garderen E, van der Poel HJ, et al. Tyrosinase gene expression in clear cell sarcoma indicates a melanocytic origin: insight from the first reported canine case. APMIS 1999;107(11):982–8.

97. Ramos-Vara JA, Beissenherz ME, Miller MA, et al. Retrospective study of 338 canine oral melanomas with clinical, histologic, and immunohistochemical review of 129 cases. Vet Pathol 2000;37(6):597–608.

98. Ramos-Vara JA, Miller MA. Immunohistochemical identification of canine melanocytic neoplasms with antibodies to melanocytic antigen PNL2 and tyrosinase: comparison with Melan A. Vet Pathol 2011;48(2):443–50.

99. de Vries TJ, Smeets M, de GR, et al. Expression of gp100, MART-1, tyrosinase, and S100 in paraffin-embedded primary melanomas and locoregional, lymph node, and visceral metastases: implications for diagnosis and immunotherapy. A study conducted by the EORTC Melanoma Cooperative Group. J Pathol 2001; 193(1):13–20.

100. Gradilone A, Gazzaniga P, Ribuffo D, et al. Prognostic significance of tyrosinase expression in sentinel lymph node biopsy for ultra-thin, thin, and thick melanomas. Eur Rev Med Pharmacol Sci 2012;16(10):1367–76.

101. Liao JC, Gregor P, Wolchok JD, et al. Vaccination with human tyrosinase DNA induces antibody responses in dogs with advanced melanoma. Cancer Immun 2006;6:8.

102. Goubier A, Fuhrmann L, Forest L, et al. Superiority of needle-free transdermal plasmid delivery for the induction of antigen-specific IFNgamma T cell responses in the dog. Vaccine 2008;26:2186–90.

103. Grosenbaugh DA, Leard AT, Bergman PJ, et al. Safety and efficacy of a xenogeneic DNA vaccine encoding for human tyrosinase as adjunctive treatment for oral malignant melanoma in dogs following surgical excision of the primary tumor. Am J Vet Res 2011;72(12):1631–8.

104. Herzog A, Buchholz J, Ruess-Melzer K, et al. Concurrent irradiation and DNA tumor vaccination in canine oral malignant melanoma: a pilot study. Schweiz Arch Tierheilkd 2013;155(2):135–42 [in German].

105. Ottnod JM, Smedley RC, Walshaw R, et al. A retrospective analysis of the efficacy of Oncept vaccine for the adjunct treatment of canine oral malignant melanoma. Vet Comp Oncol 2013;11(3):219–29.

106. Wolchok JD, Yuan J, Houghton AN, et al. Safety and immunogenicity of tyrosinase DNA vaccines in patients with melanoma. Mol Ther 2007;15:2044–50.

107. Perales MA, Yuan J, Powel S, et al. Phase I/II study of GM-CSF DNA as an adjuvant for a multipeptide cancer vaccine in patients with advanced melanoma. Mol Ther 2008;16:2022–9.

108. Yuan J, Ku GY, Gallardo HF, et al. Safety and immunogenicity of a human and mouse gp100 DNA vaccine in a phase I trial of patients with melanoma. Cancer Immun 2009;9:5.

109. Manley CA, Leibman NF, Wolchok JD, et al. Xenogeneic murine tyrosinase DNA vaccine for malignant melanoma of the digit of dogs. J Vet Intern Med 2011; 25(1):94–9.

110. Phillips JC, Blackford JT, Lembcke LM, et al. Evaluation of needle-free injection devices for intramuscular vaccination in horses. J Equine Vet Sci 2011;31: 738–43.

111. Peggs KS, Quezada SA, Korman AJ, et al. Principles and use of anti-CTLA4 antibody in human cancer immunotherapy. Curr Opin Immunol 2006;18(2):206–13.

112. Graves SS, Stone D, Loretz C, et al. Establishment of long-term tolerance to SRBC in dogs by recombinant canine CTLA4-Ig. Transplantation 2009;88: 317–22.

113. Biller BJ, Elmslie RE, Burnett RC, et al. Use of FoxP3 expression to identify regulatory T cells in healthy dogs and dogs with cancer. Vet Immunol Immunopathol 2007;116:69–78.

114. Horiuchi Y, Tominaga M, Ichikawa M, et al. Increase of regulatory T cells in the peripheral blood of dogs with metastatic tumors. Microbiol Immunol 2009;53: 468–74.

115. O'Neill K, Guth A, Biller B, et al. Changes in regulatory T cells in dogs with cancer and associations with tumor type. J Vet Intern Med 2009;23:875–81.

116. Sherger M, Kisseberth W, London C, et al. Identification of myeloid derived suppressor cells in the peripheral blood of tumor bearing dogs. BMC Vet Res 2012; 8:209.

117. Thamm DH. Interactions between radiation therapy and immunotherapy: the best of two worlds? Vet Comp Oncol 2006;4:189–97.

118. Walter CU, Biller BJ, Lana SE, et al. Effects of chemotherapy on immune responses in dogs with cancer. J Vet Intern Med 2006;20(2):342–7.

119. Emens LA, Jaffee EM. Leveraging the activity of tumor vaccines with cytotoxic chemotherapy. Cancer Res 2005;65(18):8059–64.

120. Wolchok JD, Kluger H, Callahan MK, et al. Nivolumab plus ipilimumab in advanced melanoma. N Engl J Med 2013;369(2):122–33.

121. Chu PY, Pan SL, Liu CH, et al. KIT gene exon 11 mutations in canine malignant melanoma. Vet J 2013;196(2):226–30.

122. Murakami A, Mori T, Sakai H, et al. Analysis of KIT expression and KIT exon 11 mutations in canine oral malignant melanomas. Vet Comp Oncol 2011;9(3): 219–24.

123. Gillard M, Cadieu E, De BC, et al. Naturally occurring melanomas in dogs as models for non-UV pathways of human melanomas. Pigment Cell Melanoma Res 2014;27(1):90–102.

124. Khanna C, London C, Vail D, et al. Guiding the optimal translation of new cancer treatments from canine to human cancer patients. Clin Cancer Res 2009;15: 5671–7.

125. Paoloni M, Khanna C. Translation of new cancer treatments from pet dogs to humans. Nat Rev Cancer 2008;8:147–56.

126. Ranieri G, Gadaleta CD, Patruno R, et al. A model of study for human cancer: spontaneous occurring tumors in dogs. Biological features and translation for new anticancer therapies. Crit Rev Oncol Hematol 2013;88(1):187–97.
127. Angstadt AY, Thayanithy V, Subramanian S, et al. A genome-wide approach to comparative oncology: high-resolution oligonucleotide aCGH of canine and human osteosarcoma pinpoints shared microaberrations. Cancer Genet 2012; 205(11):572–87.

Chemotherapy Safety in Clinical Veterinary Oncology

Shawna Klahn, DVM

KEYWORDS

- Chemotherapy • Safety • Veterinary oncology • Closed-system transfer device
- Personal protective equipment • NIOSH

KEY POINTS

- Exposure to chemotherapy occurs both at the clinic and in the pet owner's home through direct contact and environmental contamination.
- Health care workers who handle chemotherapy have measurable levels of chemotherapy in urine, mutagenicity of urine, increased DNA damage, and an increased risk of reproductive failure and cancer development.
- Multiple levels of hazard control and appropriate handling techniques must be used to minimize contamination and the risks associated with exposure.
- Oral, at-home cancer therapies carry additional management and safety concerns.
- Several states have passed laws to mandate implementation of the National Institute for Occupational Safety and Health guidelines for handling hazardous drugs; veterinary clinics that handle chemotherapy are affected by these laws.

Videos of proper donning of personal protective equipment, proper technique before, during, and following administration, and proper doffing and waste disposal accompany this article at http://www.vetsmall.theclinics.com/

HISTORY OF CHEMOTHERAPY SAFETY

Chemotherapy as a treatment of cancer in pets began in earnest in the early 1970s, a mere 25 years after the birth of human medical oncology. In 1979, a letter in *The Lancet* documented mutagenicity of the urine of nurses handling cytotoxic chemotherapy.[1] This letter sparked a new field of interest in cancer chemotherapy: chemotherapy safety for health care personnel. Studies were launched investigating the existence of exposure, routes of exposure, methods to determine and monitor exposure, and the mutation frequency, reproductive failures, and risk of cancer

---

The author has nothing to disclose.

Department of Small Animal Sciences, Virginia-Maryland Regional College of Veterinary Medicine, Virginia Tech, 205 Duck Pond Drive, Blacksburg, VA 24061, USA

E-mail address: klahn@vt.edu

Vet Clin Small Anim 44 (2014) 941–963

http://dx.doi.org/10.1016/j.cvsm.2014.05.009

vetsmall.theclinics.com

development associated with exposure. Limitations in detection methods and confounding factors such as genetic predisposition, lifestyle, level and duration of exposure, and the impact of safety measures makes interpretation and comparison of studies difficult. The mission to identify chemotherapy as an occupational hazard and determine the acceptable level of risk is complex and cost-prohibitive. To detect a 2-fold increase in the risk of cancer, it would be necessary to follow tens of thousands of exposed individuals and an equal number of nonexposed persons over a 20- to 30-year time period.[2] The consensus is that prudence is indicated; in the absence of definitive data, chemotherapy safety practice should mirror the guidelines for laboratory workers who handle hazardous drugs.

A provocative review published in 1987 gave voice to the unanswered questions of the time (**Box 1**).[2] Although 35 years of research and more than 150 publications have sought to provide answers, the strongest answer to most of them is still "maybe." The single question to which there is a definitive answer is whether veterinary oncologists should be appraised of drug-handling safety concerns. The answer is a resounding "yes." Furthermore, awareness of drug-handling safety concerns must extend beyond those that specialize in veterinary oncology.

RELEVANCE TO VETERINARY MEDICINE

In human medicine, advances in the diagnosis and treatment of cancer have led to living with cancer rather than dying from it. This paradigm shift has led to greater focus on quality of life and convenience. Cancer treatments are administered mainly within the local outpatient setting and there is an increase in the use of oral, at-home

---

Box 1
Unanswered questions regarding chemotherapy safety (1987)

- Does low-level exposure to cytotoxic agents on a long-term basis lead to significant absorption?
- Does low-level exposure cause acute or long-term side effects?
- Should personnel actively attempting to conceive handle cytotoxic agents?
- Are pharmacists at risk in packaging oral cytotoxic agents through aerosols generated during the preparation process?
- Do all antineoplastic agents pose a risk?
- Which pose the greatest risk?
- Do sweat tears, saliva, and other body fluids contain significant amount of cytotoxic metabolites that require safety precautions?
- Does septic system disposal of excreta pose a risk to the general public?
- Do soiled linen and items not capable of being laundered pose a hazard?
- What is the safest carcinogenic waste destruction method?
- Should morticians and pathology staff handle expired patients and specimens with special precautions?
- Should veterinarian oncologists be appraised of drug handling safety concerns as they treat household pets with cytotoxic agents?
- Do these questions reflect valid concerns or are they an overreaction to what some consider an emotional issue?

Data from Miller SA. Issues in cytotoxic drug handling safety. Semin Oncol Nurs 1987;3(2):133–41.

anticancer agents. Similar trends have occurred in veterinary medicine, resulting in treatments that are administered at home or a local clinic. However, there are key differences between human and veterinary medicine regarding cancer management practices and chemotherapy safety. Human outpatient cancer clinics are staffed with medical oncologists and trained oncology nurses. Outpatient clinics must comply with the American Society of Clinical Oncology/Oncology Nursing Society (ASCO/ONS) standards for safe chemotherapy administration[3] to achieve certification in the Quality Oncology Practice Initiative Program (QOPI).[4] In veterinary medicine, chemotherapy in local practices is literally placed in the hands of general practitioners, staff, and pet owners, without any oversight to evaluate the safety of administration. A recent study identified the veterinary medicine sector as one of "primary concern" for exposure to antineoplastic drugs, with levels of exposure measuring 15 times higher than those within the human hospital setting.[5]

PROTECTION MOTIVATION THEORY AND LACK OF COMPLIANCE

Numerous guidelines, recommendations, safety standards, and consensus statements have been published in both human and veterinary medicine by national organizations such as the National Institute for Occupational Safety and Health (NIOSH),[6,7] the American Society of Clinical Oncology–Oncology Nursing Society (ASCO-ONS),[3] the American Society of Health-System Pharmacists (ASHP),[8] the European Colleges of Veterinary Internal Medicine (ECVIM),[9] and the American College of Veterinary Internal Medicine (ACVIM). In addition, multiple reviews have been published in journals that target a wide veterinary audience.[10–17] A provocative question is why compliance with safety recommendations remains inconsistent. This gap is not unique to veterinary facilities, as several studies in human medicine indicate that the level of knowledge does not heavily influence the use of safety measures in practice.[18–20] Reported barriers include factors such as inconvenience, discomfort, cost, and time. Overcoming these barriers requires motivation to protect one's health, which is influenced by an individual belief system. The Protection Motivation Theory lists 5 components, providing a theoretical framework to predict health behaviors (**Box 2**).[18] Therefore, attempts to improve the level and consistency of chemotherapy safety standards should target health care workers' motivation for self-protection. Self-efficacy is not reported to be a major hurdle, and the influence of negative factors can be overridden if the perceptions of susceptibility, severity, and the benefits of taking a health action are appropriately addressed.

Box 2
Five factors of the Protection Motivation Theory to explain health behavior

- Perceived susceptibility: the individual's perception of his chances of becoming ill

- Perceived severity of the health problem

- Perceived benefits: the benefits of taking a particular health action to reduce the threat of adverse effects

- Perceived barriers: the influence of the negative factors on the individual's health behavior

- Self-efficacy: the individual's ability and capability to perform according to the health recommendation to achieve success in health activities

Data from Ben-Ami S, Shaham J, Rabin S, et al. The influence of nurses' knowledge, attitudes, and health beliefs on their safe behavior with cytotoxic drugs in Israel. Cancer Nurs 2001;24(3):9.

STATE LEGISLATION MANDATING COMPLIANCE

A significant lack of veterinary-specific studies may partially explain reluctance to comply with chemotherapy safety practices. However, this may no longer be considered acceptable justification for substandard safety practices or a disregard for safety standards. Under the Occupational Safety and Health Act of 1970, employers are responsible for providing a safe and healthful workplace. However, guidelines published by NIOSH have not been directly enforceable, and compliance has been voluntary.

The seed of change was planted in 2008, when Sue Crump, a Seattle pharmacist, was diagnosed with pancreatic cancer. Crump had been exposed to chemotherapy during her long career working with hazardous drugs. In 2010, a story on the dangers of hazardous drugs was published in the *Seattle Times*. In April of 2011, the State of Washington became the first to pass legislation mandating compliance with NIOSH guidelines.[21–24] A similar bill was signed into law in the State of California in October of 2013[23,25]; the State of North Carolina will likely pass similar legislation in 2014.[23,26,27] These landmark laws will have an impact on the handling of chemotherapy in all facilities, including veterinary practices. The Washington State Veterinary Medical Association has worked closely with the state Department of Labor and Industry to facilitate implementation of the guidelines.[28] The complex field of chemotherapy safety has not been fully embraced by veterinary medical practice. However, inevitably, a higher degree of incorporation will be demanded. Chemotherapy safety can easily be integrated alongside foundational cancer management skills during the training of future technical staff, clinicians, and specialists.

DEFINING EXPOSURE AND HEALTH RISK: A METHOD TO THE MADNESS

There are 3 categories for documenting exposure to chemotherapy (**Fig. 1**). Environmental monitoring (EM) uses wipe-sampling methods to detect the drug in the environment. Limitations of EM are that the sampling and assay methods are drug-dependent, samples are taken from a representative area, 100% recovery is assumed, and results do not directly translate into internalization and health risk associated with exposure. However, EM is useful in determining potential routes of exposure, identifying persons who may be at risk of exposure, and evaluating efficacy of engineering control methods.

Biological monitoring (BM) involves sampling of bodily fluids and detection of the drug and its metabolites, and/or demonstration of activity of the drug by mutagenicity assays. BM provides a better estimation of internal exposure, and is useful in identifying persons who may benefit from the use of safety precautions. However, the results of BM studies imply, but do not demonstrate, that internalization of the drug carries any impact or ultimate risks to health.

Biological effect monitoring (BEM) methods focus on evaluation of markers in biological samples as a result of exposure to proven or suspected carcinogens. BEM techniques provide an assessment of ultimate health risks, typically through demonstration of genotoxicity within easily sampled cells, which act as surrogates for the target organ or tissue. BEM are widely accepted as hazard assessment tools to define the mutagenic or carcinogenic potential of chemicals.[29] Increased levels of BEM biomarkers likely reflect a potential for increased risk of developing cancer, either directly or through increased susceptibility to damage by cocarcinogens.

The biomarkers most frequently used are cytogenetic markers such as DNA adducts, micronuclei (MN), chromosomal aberrations (CA), sister-chromatid exchanges (SCE), and cells with a high frequency of SCE (HFC). DNA adducts give rise to damage in the DNA, such as strand breaks and cross-links, which can be visualized using the

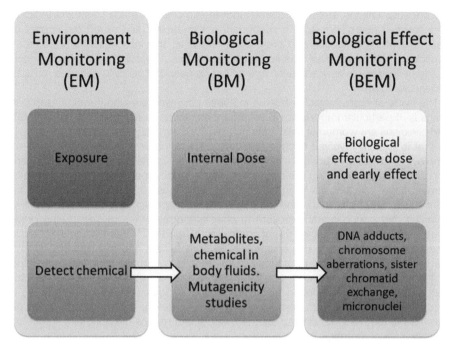

Fig. 1. Monitoring of exposure.

comet assay. The comet assay involves electrophoresis of DNA, with damaged DNA migrating toward the anode, giving a comet-like appearance to the stained gel. The amount of DNA quantified within the tail by intensity or length is directly proportional to the amount of DNA damage.[30] SCE are a result of homologous exchanges between sister chromatids, assumed to be a consequence of errors in DNA replication, indicating that the DNA has been damaged and repaired. HFC is defined as the percentage of cells with a high frequency of SCE, typically referenced against the pooled data of a control population used as a threshold value. Limitations of the assay, in which underestimation of damage may occur, are due to other DNA repair mechanisms that may not be measured.

All BEM markers indicate an early biological effect. However, DNA adducts, SCE, and HFC are reversible, decline rapidly within a few weeks, and potentially have no further consequences. CA and MN are an indication of permanent genetic damage resulting from chromosome breakage. MN are small nuclear-like bodies, containing a chromosomal fragment or whole chromosome, that have become separated from the main nucleus during cell division. CA are a result of chromosome breakage or breakage and rejoining within or between chromosomes. Levels of CA and MN in patients with cancer treated with cytostatic drugs have been constant and persistent for 2 to 10 years following cessation of therapy. There are various types of CA, including translocations, which are stable in lymphocytes and persist through cell division. Thus, translocation analysis can provide information on past and chronic exposures.[29]

EVIDENCE OF HEALTH RISK: BIOLOGICAL EFFECT MONITORING AND REPRODUCTIVE CONCERNS

The purpose of BEM is to provide an assessment of ultimate health risks of handling chemotherapy, specifically for determining the risk for development of cancer and reproductive failures. Data for patients undergoing chemotherapy treatment indicate an increased risk of developing secondary malignancies, and report the impact of treatment on reproduction and pregnancy. However, this information is not directly applicable to occupational chemotherapy exposure. The full impact of daily, low-dosage exposure to antineoplastic agents over a period of years to decades remains largely unknown.

The issue of reproductive concerns in health care workers who handle hazardous drugs is of particular importance in veterinary medicine, as a large proportion of staff and clinicians are women of child-bearing age. Furthermore, simply working in a facility that is actively involved in chemotherapy preparation or administration places all employees at risk of exposure owing to environmental contamination. Although there is no consensus regarding the impact of veterinary occupational exposure, several studies have investigated infertility and pregnancy loss in human medicine. Data from nearly 3000 pharmacy and nursing staff and approximately 7400 pregnancies revealed that occupational exposure to chemotherapy by the mother during pregnancy resulted in an increased risk of spontaneous abortion.[31] Handling antineoplastic drugs also increased the risk of infertility in both female and male pharmacy and nursing staff. A meta-analysis of studies published between 1966 and 2004 identified 7 studies suitable for statistical pooling,[32] and indicated an increased risk of spontaneous abortions in association with occupational exposure to chemotherapy. As a result, health care workers who are trying to conceive or are pregnant should be informed of the risks and offered alternative duties to reduce the potential of adverse reproductive outcomes.

There are few BEM studies evaluating conventional biomarkers in the human literature, and none involving health care workers in the United States or Canada. There are no BEM studies in veterinary medicine. The key BEM studies in the human literature are summarized in **Table 1**. The use of engineering controls and personal protective equipment (PPE) is inconsistently reported, although studies that evaluated the impact of PPE and use of a vertical flow cabinet suggest that biomarker levels are decreased in protected workers in comparison with those without the same level of protection.[29,33] Despite the use of PPE, all but one study reported a significant increase in genotoxicity when compared with the nonexposed control population. This finding suggests that PPE alone or in combination with a vertical flow cabinet is not sufficient to provide protection against exposure. Additional levels of hazard control are necessary to reduce the risk to the same level of risk as for any other occupation.

The single study involving health care workers in the United States evaluated signature chromosome abnormalities of chromosomes 5, 7, and 11.[34] In patients who have undergone chemotherapy treatment, nonrandom arrangements have been described in those later diagnosed with therapy-related myelodysplastic syndrome and therapy-related acute myeloid leukemia.[35] The 63 exposed subjects were involved in preparation, administration, or patient care, and were stratified into high-exposure and low-exposure groups based on the number of events in the 6-week study period. The 46 individuals in the control population were age-matched and gender-matched workers in nursing or pharmacy, but not directly involved in handling of chemotherapy. Safe handling practices included preparation in a biological safety cabinet (BSC), techniques minimizing aerosolization, and the use of gloves. This study reports a significantly increased frequency of structural and total abnormalities on chromosome 5 in the high-exposure group, and increased incidence rate ratios for abnormalities of chromosome 5 or 7 per 100 handling events. These effect sizes were augmented 2- to 4-fold when alkylating agent handling alone was considered. Although this study does not report genotoxicity using a conventional biomarker,

Table 1
Summary of key biological effect monitoring studies

Study Population	Control Population	Biomarker	Use of Hazard Controls	Result	Authors, Ref. Year
95 nurses from 4 different hospitals (Hungary)	Historical data (74) and industrial cohorts (34) matched for gender, age, and lifestyle	CA	All used PPE (type not reported). Differences in biosafety cabinet usage	Significant elevations in nurses working without BSC or in horizontal flow cabinet compared with nurses working in vertical flow cabinet. Significant elevations in all groups compared with historical and industrial controls	Jakab et al,[33] 2011
20 nurses (Turkey)	18 gender- and age-matched controls	CA	Not reported	2.5-fold increase in CA compared with population control level	Burgaz et al,[44] 2002
25 nurses and 5 pharmacy employees (Italy)	30 healthy subjects from same hospital matched for gender, age, and lifestyle	Comet assay: PBL and buccal cells	Gloves, gowns, masks, caps, goggles	Elevations in pharmacy technicians and day nurses via buccal cells. Elevations in pharmacy technicians via lymphocytes. No statistical significance detected	Ursini et al,[83] 2006
60 nurses (South India)	60 age- and gender-matched controls	Whole blood comet assay and MN; buccal cell MN	Routine working conditions; not reported	Significant increase in all biomarkers compared with controls	Rekhadevi et al,[84] 2007
57 female nurses in 3 different hospitals who had handled HDs in last 6 mo (Japan)	46 clerks and 64 nurses who had not handled HDs in last 6 mo. All from same hospitals, gender-matched	Comet assay: PBL	Data collected but not reported	Increased tail length in all nurses compared with clerks. No significant difference between nurse groups	Sasaki et al,[85] 2008
402 HCWs in 22 different hospitals (Croatia)	Previously reported values in healthy population	SCE and HFC in PBL	Gloves, gowns, caps, eye protection, masks	Significant elevation in both biomarkers compared with controls	Kopjar et al,[86] 2009
52 HCWs (Italy)	52 healthy subjects	Comet assay: PBL	80% wore gloves and masks	Statistically significant elevation in HCW biomarker compared with controls. Decreased values in protected HCWs compared with those without PPE	Villarini et al,[30] 2011

Abbreviations: BSC, biological safety cabinet; CA, chromosomal aberrations; HCW, health care worker; HD, hazardous drug; HFC, high-frequency (of SCE) cells; MN, micronuclei; PBL, peripheral blood lymphocytes; PPE, personal protective equipment; SCE, sister-chromatid exchanges.
Data from Refs.[30,33,44,83–86]

the findings raise concerns that chronic occupational exposure to chemotherapy may result in an increased risk of developing cancer.

ROUTES OF EXPOSURE AND PERSONS AT RISK: ENVIRONMENTAL AND BIOLOGICAL MONITORING

Documentation of environmental contamination of chemotherapy forms the basis for identifying routes of exposure and persons at risk for exposure. Each phase of contact with the drug has been evaluated as a possible exposure point (**Fig. 2**). The most common routes of exposure to chemotherapy are dermal, inhalation, and ingestion. Dermal and ingestion likely represent the most significant routes of exposure because of widespread environmental contamination and cross-contamination, and because most chemotherapy agents do not vaporize at room temperature.[36]

Many studies have documented environmental contamination in human and veterinary oncology centers.[5,37–41] Areas used to prepare and administer chemotherapy have been shown to be contaminated.[37,38,40,42] The urine of health care workers involved in the preparation and administration of chemotherapy have measurable urine levels of chemotherapy.[43–45] Contamination has been found on used PPE,[38,46] door handles of the pharmacy,[47] and the outside of drug vials,[38,48] indicating that cross-contamination occurs during the preparation and administration processes through improper technique.

Contamination has also been documented on vials that are received directly from the manufacturer, despite lack of breakage or leakage,[49–51] so persons involved in receipt of the shipments are at risk of exposure. Improper disposal of items used during treatment and patient care may also result in contamination of waste containers and potential exposure to cleaning staff.[40] In several studies, clinic areas away from chemotherapy preparation and administration sites have also been contaminated,

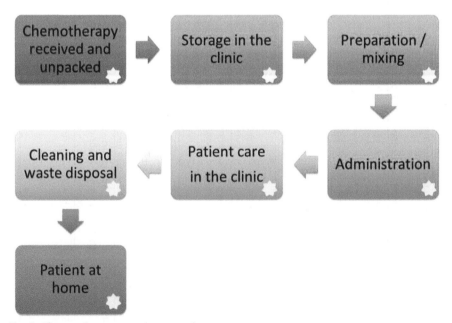

Fig. 2. Phases of contact and routes of exposure.

such as computers and floors.[38,40] It cannot be assumed that persons not directly involved in handling hazardous drugs are removed from the risk of exposure. In fact, chemotherapy has been detected in the urine of such workers.[41] In addition, the degree of contamination has not been correlated with the number of drugs and extent of use, so low-caseload facilities may not have a lower exposure risk.[40]

Once treated, the patient becomes the source of contamination, exposing caretakers and cleaning staff through contaminated laundry, excreta, and patient housing areas, with toilets demonstrating a high level of contamination.[5,37,40,52] Consequently, there have been concerns regarding the impact on wastewater and surface water.[53] Furthermore, contamination has been documented in patients' homes, and chemotherapy has been found in family members' urine following outpatient treatment.[54]

The time period for excretion of chemotherapy drugs varies depending on the agent, route of administration, and species. Although most of the available data used in veterinary medicine has been extrapolated from human studies (**Table 2**), recent studies have evaluated the levels of chemotherapy in the urine and serum in dogs following treatment with 4 commonly used drugs in veterinary medicine.[55–57] In a separate study, platinum excretion in dogs was documented for up to 21 days following treatment.[58]

Based on the potential points of exposure and the patient as a source of contamination, the list of persons at risk of chemotherapy exposure expands to include those who are more distant from the treatment process, such as workers off-site and members of the patient's household (**Table 3**). Therefore, controlling environmental contamination through engineering and administrative methods is critical.

Table 2
Detectable chemotherapy drugs in excretory products after administration

Cytotoxic Drug	Major Route of Excretion[87]	Excretory Products Tested in Studies	Period of Detection After Administration (d)	Species Studied
Parenteral agents	Agent-dependent	Not indicated	2	Human[3,6]
Oral agents		Not indicated	5–7	Human[75]
5-Fluorouracil	Urine	Urine of patient and family members	≥2	Human[54]
Carboplatin	Urine	Urine, feces, saliva, sebum, cerumen	21	Canine[58]
Chlorambucil	Urine	Not indicated	2	Human[9]
Cisplatin	Urine	Not indicated	8	Human[9]
Cyclophosphamide	Urine	Urine, serum	4, <7	Canine[56,57]
Cyclophosphamide		Urine of patient and family members	≥2	Human[54]
Cytarabine	Urine	Not indicated	3	Human[9]
Doxorubicin	Urine, feces	Urine, serum	21, <7	Canine[56,57]
Gemcitabine	Urine	Not indicated	7	Human[9]
Lomustine	Urine	Not indicated	3	Human[9]
Mitoxantrone	Feces	Not indicated	8	Human[9]
Vincristine	Bile, feces	Urine, serum	3, <7	Canine[56,57]
Vinblastine	Bile, feces	Urine, serum	7, <7	Canine[56,57]

Data from Refs.[3,6,9,54,56–58,75]

Table 3
Persons at risk of exposure to chemotherapy

Persons at Risk	Phase of Process	Route of Exposure
Inventory personnel	Shipment receipt	Contaminated and/or leaking vials
All staff/personnel	Storage	Cross-contamination of vials and environment
All staff/personnel	Preparation	Spills, inhalation, dermal, and environment
All staff/personnel	Administration	Spills, inhalation, dermal, and environment
All staff/personnel	Patient care	Patient, contaminated housing, and patient excreta
All staff/personnel	Cleaning/waste disposal	Contaminated prep/administration areas/materials, housing area/materials, patient excreta
Pet owners/family	Patient at home	Patient, patient excreta, oral anticancer agent storage/prep/administration

HAZARD CONTROL AND RECOMMENDED HEALTH ACTIONS

Each facility will have individualized needs and requirements, and development of a Hazardous Drug Safety Program is encouraged. Assessment begins with documenting the hazardous drugs used in the facility. The NIOSH Working Group on Hazardous Drugs compiled a sample list of major hazardous drugs for the Alert published in 2004. A drug was classified as hazardous if it exhibits 1 or more of the following characteristics: carcinogenicity, teratogenicity or developmental toxicity, reproductive toxicity, organ toxicity at low doses, genotoxicity, and/or has a structure and toxicity profile that mimic existing hazardous drugs.[59] This list was updated in 2010 and again in 2012,[59] providing a sampling of the major hazardous drugs. The list is not exhaustive, quickly becomes outdated because of new drug approvals, and is intended to provide guidance for the creation of a facility-specific list as part of a hazard communication program.

Environmental, biological, and BEM studies have demonstrated that occupational exposure to chemotherapy results in internalization and genotoxic damage greater than that experienced in persons with no occupational hazardous drug handling. In radiation safety, the ALARA (As Low As Reasonably Achievable) principle is used to minimize exposure, based on the assumption that each dose of any magnitude can produce some level of detrimental effects. Procedures and engineering controls are used to achieve doses as far below specified limits as reasonable. In radiation safety, the maximum annual occupational dose limits are known. In chemotherapy safety, however, there are no recommended exposure limits, permissible exposure limits, or threshold limit values. Thus there is no established acceptable level of risk, and the only safe level of exposure to chemotherapy is zero. Typically the application of the hierarchy of hazard control is to identify the most effective method of risk reduction (**Fig. 3**). With regard to chemotherapy safety, the goal of ALARA is to achieve doses as close to zero as possible, requiring utilization of multiple levels of hazard control simultaneously.

Levels 1 and 2: Eliminate or Substitute the Hazard

The first and best strategy is to eliminate the hazard. In the management of veterinary patients with cancer, this may entail referral of the client to a practice that is equipped to handle and manage the use of hazardous drugs. Recently, the American Animal

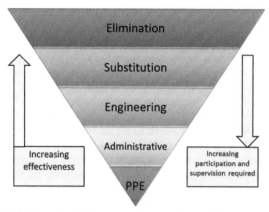

Fig. 3. Hazard control hierarchy. PPE, personal protective equipment.

Hospital Association established guidelines for the practice of veterinary dentistry.[60] According to these guidelines, "the dental health care team is obligated to practice within the scope of their respective education, training, and experience." In the practice of veterinary oncology, common sense dictates that any veterinarian administering or prescribing chemotherapy falls under similar obligations in regard of cancer management and chemotherapy safety practices. Referral to a clinician operating in a practice with multiple, concurrent methods of hazard control takes into consideration the best possible outcome for the patient, client, and workers in the referring practice.

Substitution as a hazard control method in chemotherapy safety is not applicable, as there are no safe and effective alternatives to cytotoxic drugs.

Level 3: Engineering Controls

If handling of chemotherapy cannot be eliminated from practice, the next most effective method of hazard control is implementation of engineering controls, which are physical changes to the work area or process that enclose, isolate, or redirect the hazard. Examples include the use of a ventilated cabinet or isolator, a closed-system transfer device, and separate areas dedicated to preparation, administration, and patient care.

Vertical laminar flow hoods (BSCs) and isolators are designed to protect the worker by controlling emission of airborne contaminants and containment of spills during preparation. A 2001 study evaluated genotoxicity in 3 groups of nurses: those who prepared cytostatic drugs without a biosafety cabinet, those who used a horizontal laminar flow cabinet, and those who used a vertical laminar flow biosafety cabinet.[33] Significantly higher frequency of CA in nurses lacking appropriate safety equipment were found in comparison with nurses who prepared drugs within a vertical laminar flow cabinet. All 3 groups, however, had higher levels compared with historical and industrial control populations. Therefore, use of appropriate ventilated cabinets in the preparation of cytostatic drugs reduces anticipated exposure, but is not sufficient as the sole control method. Different classes and types of BSCs exist. A brief overview and requirements to aid in BSC selection can be found in published guidelines and state legislation.[6,8,17,24]

Closed-system transfer devices (CSTD) are the only devices specifically designed to protect health care workers from occupational exposure to hazardous drugs. A CSTD mechanically prevents the transfer of environmental contaminants into the system and the escape of hazardous drugs or vapor out of the system.[6] Significant reduction in environmental contamination following implementation of a CSTD has been reported in multiple studies, including one veterinary study.[39–41,47,61,62] Several CSTDs are currently on the market and appear to be competent under multiple-test assessment.[63] A CSTD is intended to be used in conjunction with a BSC, and according to both NIOSH and ASHP guidelines is not a substitute for a ventilated cabinet.[6,8] Potential barriers to implementation of a CSTD are the cost and time added to each chemotherapy treatment. A recent review refers to the use of a CSTD as the same as the use of lead aprons in radiology, and should be simply viewed as a "cost of doing business."[64] Addressing the time factor, one study found that PhaSeal use during preparation added an additional hour per 100 samples.[65] However, the actual time was likely much less, as the time necessary for decontamination was not taken into account (necessary 24 times using standard preparation technique vs 3 times when using PhaSeal). A study evaluating the cost-saving capacity of using PhaSeal was conducted in 2012.[66] The investigators evaluated the use of the PhaSeal system in 25 agents with a chemical stability of at least 48 hours that were supplied as single-use vials. These agents maintained sterility for 7 days, suggesting that the unused portion of these vials could be salvaged. The mean potential drug wastage was 57%, and nearly half of the potential wastage was avoided. The actual saving in costs over a 50-day period was approximately $100,000. Annually, this offset the cost of the CSTD system by a factor of 7, and has the added benefit of decreased environmental contamination in the form of chemotherapy waste. Although the typical veterinary facility would not expect a similar level of chemotherapy preparation volume, a great potential exists for positive impact and offset of the financial investment of implementing the use of a CSTD.

The final method of isolating or enclosing a hazard is to dedicate separate spaces for preparation, administration, and patient care. This approach limits the potential for environmental and cross-contamination and, thus, the personnel exposed. Descriptions, recommendations, and requirements for dedicated areas have been published elsewhere,[6–8] and are listed in the ACVIM Consensus Statement for chemotherapy safety in veterinary practice.

Level 4: Administrative Controls

Administrative controls do not involve physical changes, but instead are work practices: use of warning signs (**Figs. 4** and **5**), staff training, written operating procedures, safety and health rules, and use of the buddy system (**Fig. 6**). Administrative controls are considered less effective than engineering controls, and require a higher level of participation and supervision. However, their importance should not be underestimated. Work practices not only reduce environmental contamination, but protect the worker and are integral parts of each step of the chemotherapy process. Several work practices have been associated with decreased environmental contamination, including priming of the intravenous tubing with drug-free solution by the pharmacy personnel during preparation, rinsing the tubing with a drug-free solution after administration, and the use of a transport bag or tray (**Fig. 7**).[40] Other work practices include batching of preparation and administration to reduce cross-contamination between events, preparing materials before beginning the procedure (**Fig. 8**), proper donning of PPE (Video 1), proper technique before, during, and following administration (Videos 2–4), proper doffing of PPE (Video 5), use of a chemotherapy mat (**Fig. 9**), using the transport bag to collect contaminated items during administration, and use of clearly labeled waste bins with a foot-pedal operated lid placed near the preparation, administration, and patient care sites (**Fig. 10**). Only persons who have been trained

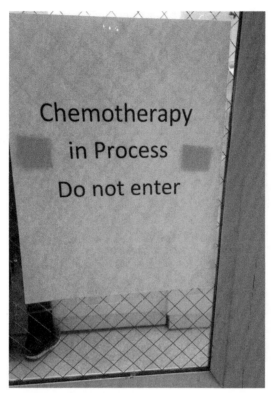

Fig. 4. Chemotherapy in process warning sign.

and assessed for proper technique should be allowed to prepare or administer chemotherapy.

Identification of an area or chemical that is hazardous can help protect persons from inadvertent exposure. The Occupational Safety and Health Administration Hazard Communication Standard (HCS) was recently updated[67] and will align with the Globally Harmonized System of Classifying and Labeling Chemicals. Full compliance with HCS is required by June 1, 2016 (see the OSHA Web site).

Disposal of chemotherapy waste is not only a source and route of exposure but is also a management concern for practices that choose to prepare and administer chemotherapy. State-specific regulations for disposal of hazardous drug waste can be found on the Environmental Protection Agency Web site.[68]

Despite improved protection and use of hazard controls, contamination occurs. Therefore, procedures for effective and efficient cleaning and decontamination, including how to respond in the event of a spill, must be in place. Several studies have been published evaluating cleaning techniques.[51,69–71] There is no one single agent that is effective in eliminating or deactivating all drugs, including bleach.[47] The combination of 2 successive steps using different agents during cleaning appears to be superior over one agent followed by application of ethanol or isopropyl alcohol.[70] A recent study assessed the availability of spill procedures for 65 antineoplastic drugs that are commonly prepared.[72] Resources used were those available to health care workers who may encounter a spill, such as the material safety data sheet, package insert, and the drug information department of the manufacturer. For most drugs,

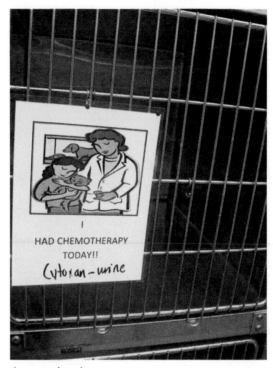

Fig. 5. Patient housing warning sign.

no reference for spill management was available. Therefore, the user must identify counteragents, if available, and develop cleaning and decontamination protocols based on knowledge of the specific drugs used. The persons directly involved in chemotherapy preparation and administration must be aware of these protocols, and trained in proper techniques for self-protection and prevention of exacerbation of the contamination.

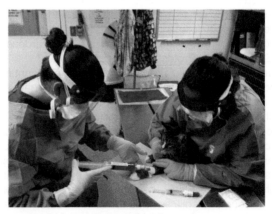

Fig. 6. Chemotherapy should be administered by 2 people.

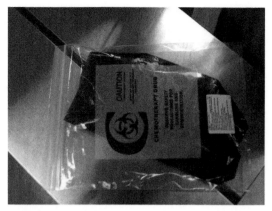

Fig. 7. Chemotherapy transport bag.

Level 5: Personal Protective Equipment

According to the OSHA, relying on PPE is a last line of defense when providing a safe and healthful workplace. Though important, the use of PPE represents the lowest effective level of protection on the hierarchy of hazard control. A recent study reported a decrease in BEM via the comet assay in workers who used PPE in comparison with workers who had insufficient protection.[29] The recommendations for PPE have been

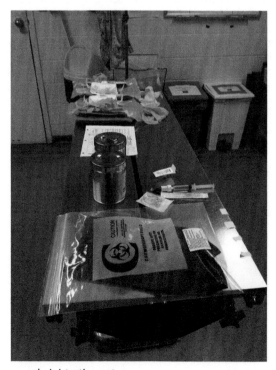

Fig. 8. Chemotherapy administration setup.

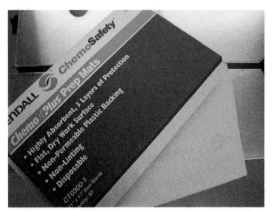

Fig. 9. Chemotherapy mat.

extensively reviewed elsewhere,[6–15,17] and include the use of chemotherapy-approved gloves (**Fig. 11**), a lint-free, low-permeability, back-closure, long-sleeved gown, a fit-tested minimum N95 respirator, and a full face shield (**Fig. 12**).

SAFE HANDLING AND ADMINISTRATION OF ORAL ANTICANCER AGENTS

The use of oral chemotherapy in human medicine is on the increase. Nearly 25% of new drugs will be orally administered agents, in part attributable to the development of targeted therapies.[3] Patient convenience also plays a role; 90% of patients with incurable cancer undergoing palliative care prefer oral administration.[73] Other advantages over intravenous administration include flexible timing and location of administration, more prolonged drug exposure, reduction in travel costs, and perception of a better quality of life. However, convenience may be lost owing to increased monitoring, daily administration, or a complex dosing schedule. There is also a misconception that oral anticancer agents are safer, although the risk for toxicity and harm is similar to that of parenteral agents. The use of oral anticancer agents may also compromise safety and result in medication errors, contamination, and inadvertent exposure to other individuals. In a review of nearly 1400 medical records, nearly

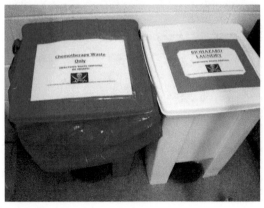

Fig. 10. Biohazard waste bins.

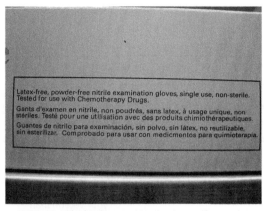

Fig. 11. Chemotherapy-approved gloves.

20% of pediatric visits had a medication error compared with 7% of adult visits, owing to high error rates in home administration.[74]

The recent addition of 2 tyrosine kinase inhibitors and the popularity of metronomic chemotherapy protocols have increased the use and availability of oral anticancer agents for veterinary clients. As many canine and feline cancers are incurable, treatments are considered palliative, and many pet owners would choose oral at-home treatment over intravenous administration if the option was available. In addition, there are parallels with human pediatric oncology, in that a caregiver is responsible for acquisition, administration, and reporting of adverse events to the physician. Typically multiple caregivers are involved, which can lead to miscommunications resulting in unsafe handling of chemotherapy at home, underdosing or overdosing, and discrepancies in reporting potential side effects. The veterinary team has a significant obligation to ensure safe handling of chemotherapy at home, although the ultimate responsibility lies with the pet owner. Many emerging issues surrounding oral anticancer agents also have implications in veterinary medicine.[73–82] The 2013 updated ASCO/ONS Chemotherapy Administration Safety Standards includes safe administration and management of oral chemotherapy, along with standards addressing chart

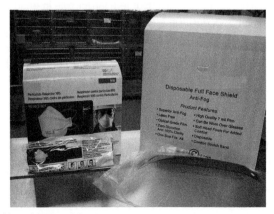

Fig. 12. Face shield and N95 respirator.

Table 4
General safe handling recommendations for pet owners

Dos	Don'ts
Review label for correct drug and dosing	Store medication with your medications, near food, or where accessible by children
Wear gloves when unpacking shipments from a compounding or mail-order pharmacy	Assume that oral chemotherapy is safer than intravenous chemotherapy
Store medication under conditions as directed by your veterinarian	Crush, split, or allow your pet to chew tablets
Wear gloves when administering medication, wash hands before and after administration	Open capsules
Report any overdosing immediately	Skip or double-up on doses unless instructed by your veterinarian
Minimize the number of people coming into contact with the medication	Modify or alter the dose or schedule without consulting with your veterinarian
Wear gloves when handling excreta	
Wash bedding separately	
Return damaged or unused medication to your veterinarian for disposal	
Keep a medication log or journal to document the administration day(s) and adverse events	

Adapted from Goodin S, Griffith N, Chen B, et al. Safe handling of oral chemotherapeutic agents in clinical practice: recommendations from an international pharmacy panel. J Oncol Pract 2011;7(1):10.

documentation, prescription requirements, and that patients should be educated regarding the storage, handling, preparation, administration, and disposal of chemotherapy. The standards are general, as many of these components will be drug-specific. The clinician and the veterinary care team must be appropriately trained and knowledgable of recommendations for prescribed chemotherapy drugs.

An international panel of pharmacists established general oral chemotherapy safe handling precautions during a review of existing guidelines.[78] The panel compiled recommendations targeting manufacturers/distributors, the health care providers, and patients/caregivers. The caregiver will assume a larger role in ensuring safe handling during all phases of contact with the anticancer agent, from receipt of the package, transport/storage, administration, and handling of excreta/soiled items (**Table 4**). Open communication regarding the potential harm and safety precautions, along with a clear understanding of the responsibilities of each of the parties involved, can help to ensure safe handling of oral chemotherapy at home and improve patients' quality of life and outcomes.

SUMMARY

Exposure to chemotherapy is a health hazard for all personnel in facilities that store, prepare, or administer antineoplastic agents. Exposure extends beyond the clinic walls to affect the patient's home and family through excreted products and the increasing use of oral at-home anticancer agents. Practical and prescriptive reviews of safe-handling guidelines are readily available, yet implementation of recommendations and guidelines is inconsistent. In this article, the published data on exposure and potential health risks is reviewed, in addition to the benefits of chemotherapy safety precautions, with the goal of increasing motivation for self-protection within the clinical veterinary oncology profession. Motivation is also provided through an increased awareness of the mandated recommendations and implications of recent state legislation, which is expected to have a significant impact on cancer management in veterinary medicine. Chemotherapy safety is an emerging field in the clinical practice of veterinary oncology, and as a community there is a need to adopt safe practices to maintain the health of staff, clients, patients, and the profession.

SUPPLEMENTARY DATA

Supplementary data related to this article can be found online at http://dx.doi.org/10.1016/j.cvsm.2014.05.009.

REFERENCES

1. Falck K, Grohn P, Sorsa M, et al. Mutagenicity in urine of nurses handling cytostatic drugs. Lancet 1979;1(8128):1250–1.
2. Miller SA. Issues in cytotoxic drug handling safety. Semin Oncol Nurs 1987;3(2):133–41.
3. Neuss MN, Polovich M, McNiff K, et al. 2013 updated American Society of Clinical Oncology/Oncology Nursing Society Chemotherapy Administration safety standards including standards for the safe administration and management of oral chemotherapy. J Oncol Pract 2013;9(2 Suppl):5s–13s.
4. Gilmore TR, Schulmeister L, Jacobson JO. Quality oncology practice initiative certification program: measuring implementation of chemotherapy administration safety standards in the outpatient oncology setting. J Oncol Pract 2013;9(2 Suppl):14s–8s.
5. Meijster T, Fransman W, Veldhof R, et al. Exposure to antineoplastic drugs outside the hospital environment. Ann Occup Hyg 2006;50(7):657–64.
6. NIOSH. NIOSH alert: preventing occupational exposures to antineoplastic and other hazardous drugs in health care settings. National Institute Occupational Safety Health 2004;2004(165):58.
7. NIOSH. Safe handling of hazardous drugs for veterinary healthcare workers. National Institute Occupational Safety Health 2010;2010(150):4.
8. American Society of Health-System Pharmacists. ASHP guidelines on handling hazardous drugs. Am J Health Syst Pharm 2006;63:21.
9. ECVIM. Preventing occupational and environmental exposure to cytotoxic drugs in veterinary medicine. In: European College of Veterinary Internal Medicine - Companion Animals, editor. Europe: 2007. p. 31. Available online at ecvim.org.
10. Lucroy MD. Chemotherapy safety in veterinary practice: hazardous drug preparation. Compendium 2001;23(10):6.
11. Lucroy MD. Chemotherapy in veterinary practice: hazardous drug administration. Compendium 2002;24(2):7.
12. Takada S. Principles of chemotherapy safety procedures. Clin Tech Small Anim Pract 2003;18(2):2.
13. Hayes A. Safe use of anticancer chemotherapy in small animal practice. In Pract 2005;27:10.
14. Fielding SL, Lacroix C. Chemotherapy safety in small animal practice. National Association of Veterinary Technicians in America 2009;Fall:6.
15. MacDonald V. Chemotherapy: managing side effects and safe handling. Can Vet J 2009;50:4.

16. Royer NS. Section C: safe handling of chemotherapy drugs. In: Henry CJ, Higginbotham ML, editors. Cancer management in small animal practice, vol. 1. Maryland Heights (MO): Saunders Elsevier; 2010. p. 107–9.

17. Flory A, Phillips B, Karriker M. Chemotherapy drug handling and safety. In: Bonagura JD, Twedt D, editors. Kirk's current veterinary therapy XV, vol. XV. St Louis (MO): Elsevier; 2014. p. 326–9.

18. Ben-Ami S, Shaham J, Rabin S, et al. The influence of nurses' knowledge, attitudes, and health beliefs on their safe behavior with cytotoxic drugs in Israel. Cancer Nurs 2001;24(3):9.

19. Polovich M, Martin S. Nurses' use of hazardous drug-handling precautions and awareness of national safety guidelines. Oncol Nurs Forum 2011;38(6):718–26.

20. Martin S, Larson E. Chemotherapy-handling practices of outpatient and office-based oncology nurses. Oncol Nurs Forum 2003;30(4):575–81.

21. Eisenberg S. NIOSH safe handling of hazardous drugs guidelines becomes state law. J Infus Nurs 2012;35(5):316–9.

22. Washington Department of Labor and Industries. Concise explanatory statement. In: WDLI, editor. WA: 2012. p. 100. Available online at: www.lni.wa.go.

23. Zock MD. Hazardous drugs and worker safety: emerging regulations. RJ Lee Group 2013; Describes Washington State law, California assembly bill (AB) 2012, and North Carolina bill (April 2019, 2013). Available at: http://www.rjlg.com/2013/04/12/hazardous-drugs-and-worker-safety-emerging-regulations/. 2013. Accessed September 13, 2013.

24. Washington State Legislature. Chapter 296-62-500. WAC General occupational health standards - hazardous drugs. 2012. Available at: http://apps.leg.wa.gov/WAC/default.aspx?cite=296-62&full=true#296-62-500. Accessed September 13, 2013.

25. Legislature Council. AB-1202 Occupational safety and health standards: hazardous drugs. In: Legislative Council, editor. 2013.

26. Carney FM. House bill 644 - prevent hazardous drug exposure. In: General Assembly of North Carolina, editor. Vol. House Bill 644. 2013.

27. Walton AM. Preventing hazardous drug exposure: N.C. House Bill 644. THE-ONC Mobile 2013; Blog Roll. Available at: http://www.theonc.org/author.asp?section_id=2765&doc_id=269431&. 2013. Accessed November 5, 2013.

28. Washington State Veterinary Medical Association. Hazardous drugs (L&I). 2013; WA Dept of Labor and Industries' hazardous drug requirements and regulations update for veterinary practices. Available at: http://www.wsvma.org/displaycommon.cfm?an=1&subarticlenbr=557. Accessed September 13, 2013.

29. van Delft JH, Baan RA, Roza L. Biological effect markers for exposure to carcinogenic compound and their relevance for risk assessment. Crit Rev Toxicol 1998;28(5):34.

30. Villarini M, Dominici L, Piccinini R, et al. Assessment of primary, oxidative and excision repaired DNA damage in hospital personnel handling antineoplastic drugs. Mutagenesis 2011;26(3):359–69.

31. Valanis B, Vollmer WM, Steele P. Occupational exposure to antineoplastic agents: self-reported miscarriages and stillbirths among nurses and pharmacists. J Occup Environ Med 1999;41(8):7.

32. Dranitsaris G, Johnston M, Poirier S, et al. Are health care providers who work with cancer drugs at an increased risk for toxic events? A systematic review and meta-analysis of the literature. J Oncol Pharm Pract 2005;11:10.

33. Jakab MG, Major J, Tompa A. Follow-up genotoxicological monitoring of nurses handling antineoplastic drugs. J Toxicol Environ Health A 2001;62(5):307–18.

34. McDiarmid MA, Oliver MS, Roth TS, et al. Chromosome 5 and 7 abnormalities in oncology personnel handling anticancer drugs. J Occup Environ Med 2010; 52(10):1028–34.
35. Pedersen-Bjergaard J, Christiansen DH, Andersen MK, et al. Causality of myelodysplasia and acute myeloid leukemia and their genetic abnormalities. Leukemia 2002;16(11):2177–84.
36. Connor TH, Shults M, Fraser MP. Determination of the vaporization of solutions of mutagenic antineoplastic agents at 23 and 37 degrees C using a desiccator technique. Mutat Res 2000;470(1):85–92.
37. Janssens T, Brouwers EE, de Vos JP, et al. Determination of platinum surface contamination in veterinary and human oncology centres using inductively coupled plasma mass spectrometry. Vet Comp Oncol 2013. [Epub ahead of print].
38. Lee ST, Tkaczuk M, Jankewicz G, et al. Surface contamination from cytotoxic chemotherapy following preparation and administration. J Pharm Pract Res 2007;37(4):6.
39. Kandel-Tschiederer B, Kessler M, Schwietzer A, et al. Reduction of workplace contamination with platinum-containing cytostatic drugs in a veterinary hospital by introduction of a closed system. Vet Rec 2010;166(26):822–5.
40. Kopp B, Schierl R, Nowak D. Evaluation of working practices and surface contamination with antineoplastic drugs in outpatient oncology health care settings. Int Arch Occup Environ Health 2013;86(1):47–55.
41. Wick C, Slawson MH, Jorgenson JA, et al. Using a closed-system protective device to reduce personnel exposure to antineoplastic agents. Am J Health Syst Pharm 2003;60(22):8.
42. Connor TH, Anderson RW, Sessink PJ, et al. Surface contamination with antineoplastic agents in six cancer treatment centers in Canada and the United States. Am J Health Syst Pharm 1999;56(14):1427–32.
43. Pethran A, Schierl R, Hauff K, et al. Uptake of antineoplastic agents in pharmacy and hospital personnel. Part I: monitoring of urinary concentrations. Int Arch Occup Environ Health 2003;76(1):5–10.
44. Burgaz S, Karahalil B, Canhi Z, et al. Assessment of genotoxic damage in nurses occupationally exposed to antineoplastics by the analysis of chromosomal aberrations. Hum Exp Toxicol 2002;21(3):129–35.
45. Fransman W, Peelen S, Hilhorst S, et al. A pooled analysis to study trends in exposure to antineoplastic drugs among nurses. Ann Occup Hyg 2007;51(3): 231–9.
46. Leboucher G, Serratrice F, Bertholle V, et al. Evaluation of platinum contamination of a hazardous drug preparation area in a hospital pharmacy. Bull Cancer 2002;89(11):949–55 [in French].
47. Clark BA, Sessink PJ. Use of a closed system drug-transfer device eliminates surface contamination with antineoplastic agents. J Oncol Pharm Pract 2013; 19(2):7.
48. Crauste-Manciet S, Sessink PJ, Ferrari S, et al. Environmental contamination with cytotoxic drugs in healthcare using positive air pressure isolators. Ann Occup Hyg 2005;49(7):619–28.
49. Favier B, Gilles L, Ardiet C, et al. External contamination of vials containing cytotoxic agents supplied by pharmaceutical manufacturers. J Oncol Pharm Pract 2003;9:7.
50. Mason HJ, Morton J, Garfitt SJ, et al. Cytotoxic drug contamination on the outside of vials delivered to a hospital pharmacy. Ann Occup Hyg 2003;47(8):5.

51. Touzin K, Bussieres JF, Langlois E, et al. Cyclophosphamide contamination observed on the external surfaces of drug vials and the efficacy of cleaning on vial contamination. Ann Occup Hyg 2008;52(8):765–71.

52. Hedmer M, Tinnerberg H, Axmon A, et al. Environmental and biological monitoring of antineoplastic drugs in four workplaces in a Swedish hospital. Int Arch Occup Environ Health 2008;81(7):899–911.

53. O'Keefe T. Cytotoxic drug contamination in hospital and municipal wastewater and its transfer to surface water. Middletown, RI: Pharma-Cycle, Inc; 2011. p. 11 Confidential.

54. Yuki M, Sekine S, Takase K, et al. Exposure of family members to antineoplastic drugs via excreta of treated cancer patients. J Oncol Pharm Pract 2013;19(3): 208–17.

55. Hamscher G, Mohring SA, Knobloch A, et al. Determination of drug residues in urine of dogs receiving anti-cancer chemotherapy by liquid chromatography-electrospray ionization- tandem mass spectrometry: is there an environmental or occupational risk? J Anal Toxicol 2010;34(3):142–8.

56. Knobloch A, Mohring SA, Eberle N, et al. Cytotoxic drug residues in urine of dogs receiving anticancer chemotherapy. J Vet Intern Med 2010;24(2):384–90.

57. Knobloch A, Mohring SA, Eberle N, et al. Drug residues in serum of dogs receiving anticancer chemotherapy. J Vet Intern Med 2010;24(2):379–83.

58. Janssens T, Brouwers EE, de Vos JP, et al. Inductively coupled plasma mass-spectrometric determination of platinum in excretion products of client-owned pet dogs. Vet Comp Oncol 2013. [Epub ahead of print].

59. NIOSH. NIOSH list of antineoplastic and other hazardous drugs in healthcare settings 2012. National Institute Occupational Safety Health 2012;2012(150):20.

60. Holmstrom SE, Bellows J, Juriga S, et al. 2013 AAHA dental care guidelines for dogs and cats. J Am Anim Hosp Assoc 2013;49(2):75–82.

61. Harrison BR, Peters BG, Bing MR. Comparison of surface contamination with cyclophosphamide and fluorouracil using a closed-system drug transfer device versus standard preparation techniques. Am J Health Syst Pharm 2006;63:9.

62. Sessink PJ, Connor TH, Jorgenson JA, et al. Reduction in surface contamination with antineoplastic drugs in 22 hospital pharmacies in the US following implementation of a closed-system drug transfer device. J Oncol Pharm Pract 2011;17(1):39–48.

63. Queruau Lamerie T, Carrez L, Decaudin B, et al. Multiple-test assessment of devices to protect healthcare workers when administering cytotoxic drugs to patients. J Oncol Pharm Pract 2012;18(2):191–200.

64. Massoomi FF. CSTDs as a cost of doing business. Pharmacy Purchasing Products Magazine 2012;5.

65. Favier B, Labrosse H, Gilles-Afchain L, et al. The PhaSeal(R) system: impact of its use on workplace contamination and duration of chemotherapy preparation. J Oncol Pharm Pract 2012;18(1):37–45.

66. Edwards MS, Solimando DA Jr, Grollman FR, et al. Cost savings realized by use of the PhaSeal(R) closed-system transfer device for preparation of antineoplastic agents. J Oncol Pharm Pract 2013;19(4):338–47.

67. US Department of Labor - Occupational Safety and Health Administration. Hazard communication standard. 2013; Aligns with the UN's globally harmonized system of classification and labelling of chemicals. Available at: https://www.osha.gov/dsg/hazcom/index.html. Accessed September 13, 2013.

68. Environmental Protection Agency. Where you live - state medical waste programs and regulations. 2013. Available at: http://www.epa.gov/osw/nonhaz/industrial/medical/programs.htm. Accessed September 13, 2013.

69. Roberts S, Khammo N, McDonnell G, et al. Studies on the decontamination of surfaces exposed to cytotoxic drugs in chemotherapy workstations. J Oncol Pharm Pract 2006;12:10.
70. Touzin K, Bussieres JF, Langlois E, et al. Pilot study comparing the efficacy of two cleaning techniques in reducing environmental contamination with cyclophosphamide. Ann Occup Hyg 2010;54(3):351–9.
71. Hon CY, Chua PP, Danyluk Q, et al. Examining factors that influence the effectiveness of cleaning antineoplastic drugs from drug preparation surfaces: a pilot study. J Oncol Pharm Pract 2013;20(3):210–6.
72. Gonzalez R, Massoomi FF. Manufacturers' recommendations for handling spilled hazardous drugs. Am J Health Syst Pharm 2010;67(23):1985–6.
73. Aisner J. Overview of the changing paradigm in cancer treatment: oral chemotherapy. Am J Health Syst Pharm 2007;64(9 Suppl 5):S4–7.
74. Walsh KE, Mazor KM, Roblin D, et al. Multisite parent-centered risk assessment to reduce pediatric oral chemotherapy errors. J Oncol Pract 2013;9(1):e1–7.
75. Griffin E. Safety considerations and safe handling of oral chemotherapy agents. Clin J Oncol Nurs 2003;7(6 Suppl):25–9.
76. Boehnke ML. Oral chemotherapy: a shifting paradigm affecting patient safety. Practice Management - HemOnc Today. 2008. Available at: http://www.healio.com/hematology-oncology/practice-management/news/print/hematology-oncology/%7Beb23b3a4-10d1-4a60-afdc-4d0724505b39%7D/oral-chemotherapy-a-shifting-paradigm-affecting-patient-safety. Accessed November 5, 2013.
77. Weingart SN, Toro J, Spencer J, et al. Medication errors involving oral chemotherapy. Cancer 2010;116(10):2455–64.
78. Goodin S, Griffith N, Chen B, et al. Safe handling of oral chemotherapeutic agents in clinical practice: recommendations from an international pharmacy panel. J Oncol Pract 2011;7(1):7–12.
79. Weingart SN, Spencer J, Buia S, et al. Medication safety of five oral chemotherapies: a proactive risk assessment. J Oncol Pract 2011;7(1):2–6.
80. Lester J. Safe handling and administration considerations of oral anticancer agents in the clinical and home setting. Clin J Oncol Nurs 2012;16(6):E192–7.
81. Bassan F, Peter F, Houbre B, et al. Adherence to oral antineoplastic agents by cancer patients: definition and literature review. Eur J Cancer Care (Engl) 2014;23(1):22–35.
82. Mathes T, Antoine SL, Pieper D, et al. Adherence enhancing interventions for oral anticancer agents: a systematic review. Cancer Treat Rev 2014;40(1):102–8.
83. Ursini CL, Cavallo D, Colombi A, et al. Evaluation of early DNA damage in healthcare workers handling antineoplastic drugs. Int Arch Occup Environ Health 2006;80(2):134–40.
84. Rekhadevi PV, Sailaja N, Chandrasekhar M, et al. Genotoxicity assessment in oncology nurses handling anti-neoplastic drugs. Mutagenesis 2007;22(6):395–401.
85. Sasaki M, Dakeishi M, Hoshi S, et al. Assessment of DNA damage in Japanese nurses handling antineoplastic drugs by the comet assay. J Occup Health 2008;50(1):7–12.
86. Kopjar N, Kasuba V, Rozgaj R, et al. The genotoxic risk in health care workers occupationally exposed to cytotoxic drugs - A comprehensive evaluation by the SCE assay. J Environ Sci Health A Tox Hazard Subst Environ Eng 2009;44:19.
87. Physicians' cancer chemotherapy drug manual. 2013 edition. Burlington (MA): Jones & Bartlett Learning; 2013.

The Role of Neutering in Cancer Development

Annette N. Smith, DVM, MS

KEYWORDS

- Neuter • Cancer • Sex hormone • Spay • Castration

KEY POINTS

- Sex hormone receptors have been found in some canine and feline tumors and implied in others through sex predilection or response to neutering.
- A few studies indicate that some tumor types may be increased in surgically altered dogs; other tumor types may be decreased in neutered animals.
- Neutering has other effects on certain behaviors, noncancerous diseases, and lifespan that may outweigh cancer risks.
- Recommendations may be different for owned animals and those in a shelter or rescue setting.
- Veterinarians and pet owners should discuss the risks and benefits of neutering for each individual.

INTRODUCTION

Sex hormones normally influence many tissues in the body, and hormone receptors are present in some canine and feline neoplasms: mammary tumors,[1–6] meningiomas,[7,8] perianal gland tumors,[9] and likely others. The administration of exogenous hormones has been associated with the development of some tumors, such as progestins in the development of canine and feline mammary tumors.[10,11] Signalment of dogs that present with certain tumor types have been associated with variable sex predilection, implying hormonal influence. Other tumors may regress or have decreased recurrence after surgical alteration.[12–14] Recently, increased scrutiny of the role of neutering in dogs on disease incidence has resulted in some interesting findings, and questions, on the potential role of sex hormones in cancer development in this species (**Table 1**).

Steroid hormones interact with cells in several ways: (1) diffusion through the cellular membrane and binding to cytoplasmic (androgen) or nuclear (estrogen) receptor proteins. The activated receptor then interacts with coregulator proteins and binds to

Department of Clinical Sciences, College of Veterinary Medicine, Bailey Small Animal Teaching Hospital, Auburn University, 1220 Wire Road, Auburn, AL 36849-5540, USA
E-mail address: smith30@auburn.edu

Vet Clin Small Anim 44 (2014) 965–975
http://dx.doi.org/10.1016/j.cvsm.2014.06.003
0195-5616/14/$ – see front matter © 2014 Elsevier Inc. All rights reserved.

Table 1 Tumor types that may be influenced by gonadectomy	
	Concerning Breeds
Tumors with increased risk post-castration	
Cardiac tumors	All
Osteosarcoma	All, purebred dogs, Rottweilers (<1 y of age at castration)
Prostatic tumors (carcinoma, adenocarcinoma, transitional cell carcinoma)	All
Transitional cell carcinoma of the urinary bladder	All
Lymphoma	All, Golden retrievers (<1 y of age at castration)
Tumors with decreased risk post-castration	
Testicular	All
Tumors with increased risk post-spay	
Cardiac tumors	All
Cardiac hemangiosarcoma	All
Osteosarcoma	Purebred dogs, Rottweilers (<1 y of age at spay)
Splenic hemangiosarcoma	All, Vizslas, Golden retrievers (>1 y of age at spay)
Mast cell tumor	All, Vizslas, Golden retrievers
Lymphoma	All
Tumors with decreased risk post-spay	
Ovarian tumors	All
Uterine tumors	All
Mammary tumors (canine, with spay before 3rd estrus)	All
Mammary tumors (feline, with spay before 3rd estrus)	All

hormone-responsive elements in the promoter regions of the DNA, which causes transcription of hormone-regulated proteins.[15] (2) Hormones may bind to receptors that interact with other transcription factors that bind to the DNA, causing indirect activation of proteins.[16] (3) Receptors may not require binding of the hormone to induce DNA transcription, rather may be activated through other growth factor pathways.[16] In humans, estrogen and testosterone affect breast and prostatic cancer growth and viability in a large percentage of patients, leading to treatments that modulate hormone levels or block their receptors.[16]

MAMMARY TUMORS

Historically, the influence of spaying on mammary tumor development has been the most well-studied veterinary sex hormone–tumor link. In sexually intact female dogs, mammary neoplasia is the most common form of cancer, based on many current large European cancer registries' databases.[17–20] Because early neutering is rare in these countries, these data help us to understand the risk in intact female dogs. Incidence of mammary tumors increases over time, which also correlates with increased exposure to female sex hormones.[17,21,22] Exogenous hormone exposure also increases the risk of tumor development.[10] Significant tumor risk occurs around 7 to

8 years of age, and increases until 11 to 13 years of age, with malignant tumors having a mean age of development around 9 to 11 years. In altered female dogs, in which female sex hormones are almost eliminated, the incidence of mammary cancer is almost eradicated by spaying before the first estrus cycle, with a 0.5% lifetime risk.[23] For a dog spayed between the first and second estrus cycle, the lifetime risk increases to 8%, and for a dog spayed after the second estrus cycle, the risk is 26%.[23] Surgical alteration between the third estrus cycle and approximately 4 years of age provides only modest protection, if any, against the development of mammary tumors.[22–25]

In cats, there are fewer data available regarding hormone-associated cancer development. A few studies have looked at the incidence of mammary tumors in intact versus spayed female cats.[26–28] In unaltered cats, mammary tumors are reported to be the third most frequent tumor type in the United States, and the most common type in European countries, although the overall incidence (25/100,000 in the United States) is less than that is reported in dogs (198/100,000 in the United States).[26–28] Increasing age increases the risk of cancer development, with significant increases occurring between 7 and 14 years.[10,26,29,30] With increasing age comes increased hormonal exposure, with intact female cats having up to a 7 times greater risk of developing mammary tumors than spayed cats.[10,26,31] Neutering before the first estrus provides a 91% risk reduction, before the second estrus an 86% risk reduction, and before the third estrus an 11% risk reduction.[31] After the age of 2 years, no benefit to surgical alteration is reported.[31] As with dogs, exogenous progestin exposure increases the incidence of mammary tumor development, more frequently benign than malignant.[10,11]

To complicate matters, an analysis of the literature on the subject of the association of neutering and canine mammary tumor development found that the evidence for the recommendation of early spay is "weak".[32] However, this is likely a reflection of the veterinary literature in general, rather than an indictment of the conclusions drawn by the multiple studies looking at the relationship between surgical alteration and mammary cancer development.

REPRODUCTIVE ORGAN TUMORS AND TUMORS TREATED BY NEUTERING

Obviously, removal of an organ does eliminate the potential for tumor development within that organ: (1) ovariohysterectomy for uterine and ovarian neoplasia and (2) castration for testicular tumors. Removal of testosterone through castration also cures greater than 90% of dogs with perianal gland tumors,[12] and testosterone production by adrenal tumors has been shown to influence the development of perianal gland tumors in female dogs.[33] Vaginal leiomyomas occur almost exclusively in intact female dogs, and ovariectomy significantly decreases the incidence of recurrence even with incomplete surgical removal of the tumor.[13,14]

Several studies have shown an increase in various prostatic carcinomas in neutered male dogs, ranging from a twice to eight times risk compared with intact male dogs.[34,35] This increase is in contrast to the androgen dependence seen in most early human prostate tumors, but may be consistent with the development of androgen-independence with disease progression.[36] However, remaining intact does not eliminate the possibility of developing prostatic carcinomas,[37] and the overall prevalence of prostatic cancer in dogs is estimated to be very low (0.2%–0.6%).[37–40]

OSTEOSARCOMA

Many studies investigating the influence of sex on appendicular osteosarcoma incidence seemed to indicate an increased risk in male dogs, although some breeds appeared to have female predilection.[41–45] A larger review of all patients with osteosarcoma (n = 1775) presenting to the Colorado State University over a 27-year period (1978–2005) did not confirm these findings, with an equal male-to-female ratio.[46] However, castration appears to have some influence, with one study reporting an increased risk of 1.3 in altered dogs compared with intact males.[47] Another study characterizing risks in purebred dogs found that neutering increased risk by approximately 1.9 times in females and 1.4 times in males when controlled for age of onset.[48] Further studies in Rottweilers (n = 683) found an increased risk of osteosarcoma development in both males and females when dogs were gonadectomized at an early age (<12 months).[49]

HEMANGIOSARCOMA

A large review of Golden Retrievers presenting to the University of California at Davis (n = 759) found that females neutered after 12 months of age (late) had a risk of being diagnosed with hemangiosarcoma 4 times greater than that of intact or females spayed early (<12 months of age).[50] No differences were found in hemangiosarcoma diagnosis based on neuter status or time of alteration in male dogs.[50] Another review assessing the role of gonadectomy on the risk of cancer development, this time in Vizslas, found that spayed females were 9 times more likely to develop hemangiosarcoma compared with intact females.[51] Females spayed early had an odds ratio (OR) of 6.0 and late-spayed females had an OR ratio of 11.5 compared with intact females.[51] Late-castrated males were 5 times more likely to develop hemangiosarcoma compared with intact males.[51] A broader study examining splenic hemangiosarcoma in multiple breeds found that spayed females were twice as likely to develop hemangiosarcoma than intact females.[52] Previous studies have also found that spayed females have a 4 times greater relative risk for the diagnosis of heart tumors compared with intact females, with the risk of cardiac hemangiosarcoma diagnosis more than 5 times greater in spayed versus intact females.[53] Neutered males also had a slightly increased risk (1.6) for developing heart tumors compared with sexually intact dogs.[53]

LYMPHOMA

A study of 15,000 canine lymphoma patients from the VMDB (Veterinary Medical Database, which collates information from multiple veterinary colleges) compared with a population of 1.2 million dogs found that intact female dogs were approximately half as likely to develop lymphoma compared with spayed females or males that were sexually altered or intact.[54] This finding is similar to findings in people, in which men are more likely to develop non-Hodgkin lymphoma (the canine counterpart) than women.[55] Other breed-specific studies have also found that spaying increases the risk of lymphoma.[50,51] However, castration was also found to be a risk factor, with alteration of both males and females increasing the risk approximately 3 to 4 times in Golden Retrievers and Vizslas.[50,51] In Golden Retrievers, specifically, early castration (before 1 year of age) increased the risk for lymphoma 3-fold, which was statistically significant.[50]

TRANSITIONAL CELL CARCINOMA

Transitional cell carcinoma of the bladder has a distinctly higher risk in females compared with males, with a 1.71 to 1.91:1 ratio of females to males.[56–58] Additionally, neutering increases risk up to 3-fold in both sexes.[58] Transitional cell carcinoma of the prostate is also more likely in castrated males, with an OR of 8.35.[35]

MAST CELL TUMORS

No consistent gender predilection has been reported for mast cell tumors in dogs,[59] but the recent study evaluating Golden Retrievers found a disparity (although not statistically significant) between the number of mast cell tumors diagnosed in altered females (2.3% in those spayed prior to one year and 5.7% spayed later) compared with intact (0%).[50] Males did not show such a disparity in mast cell tumor development between castrated and unaltered dogs.[50] When evaluating vizslas, however, investigators did find that gonadectomy in both males and females increased the risk of mast cell tumor development by twice to over fourfold, and that the tumors developed at an earlier age.[51] Another study looking at various breeds found that spayed females were at increased risk, with an OR of 4.11.[60] Interestingly, estrogen hormone receptors were not found in mast cell tumors in one study, which makes determining the role of the sex hormonal influence even less clear.[61]

THE INFLUENCE OF STERILIZATION ON LIFESPAN

Several large studies have been performed evaluating the impact of gonadectomy on overall lifespan and cause of death in dogs. Two thousand dogs submitted for necropsy revealed increasing incidence of cancer death with age (20% at 5 years, increasing to 40%–50% at ages 10–16). Neutered dogs of both sexes were older than intact dogs, although the difference was not statistically significant.[62] A 1999 study[63] evaluating 3126 general population British dogs found that the average lifespan for all dogs was approximately 11 years. Overall, cancer was the most common cause of death, with unneutered dogs dying of cancer more frequently than neutered dogs: 44.9% of intact male dogs, 34.7% of castrated males, 50.2% of intact female dogs, and 39.6% of spayed female dogs. Specific cancers were not examined. Spayed females lived longest (statistically significant) when all causes of death were considered, with an average age of 12 years, but for dogs dying of natural causes (only 8% of the population studied), intact females lived longest, with an average age of slightly over 13 years (not statistically significant). Males, both neutered and intact, lived approximately 11 years when considering all causes of death, whereas those dying of natural causes lived approximately 12 years. In both groups, intact males lived on average 3 months longer than their castrated counterparts (no statistical difference).

In American dogs, one investigator found that in more than 40,000 subjects, an average of 7.9 versus 9.4-year lifespan was found in intact versus gonadectomized dogs. Females benefitted from sterilization more than males, with a 26% increase in life expectancy and 14% increase, respectively. However, neutered dogs were more likely to die of cancer (and immune-mediated disease), whereas they were less likely to die of causes such as degenerative disease, vascular disease, infections, or trauma. Although overall risk of cancer appeared to be increased in sterilized dogs, specific cancer types were more likely to occur: transitional cell carcinoma, osteosarcoma, lymphoma, and mast cell tumors. Mammary tumors were less likely, and melanoma, squamous cell carcinoma, and prostate cancer did not appear to be affected by neutering.[64]

The previous patients were from a veterinary teaching hospital database (Veterinary Medical Database), but the results appear to be consistent when looking at a more general American population. In the 2013 Banfield report (2.2 million dogs; 460,000 cats),[65] the average lifespan of dogs was 11 years, with spayed dogs living 11.6 years compared with unspayed dogs living 9.5 years, a 23% difference. Castrated males lived 18% longer with an average lifespan of 11.1 years compared with uncastrated with a lifespan of 9.5 years. Similarly, altered cats lived longer. Overall average survival was 12.1 years, with spayed females living an average of 13.1 years, and unspayed 9.5 years, a 39% increase. Castrated cats lived 62% longer, an average of 11.8 years compared with an average of 7.5 years for intact male cats. Unaltered dogs and cats were 2 to 4 times more likely to present for trauma by being hit by a car or bitten by another animal.

In contrast, the study examining Vizslas did not find an increase in lifespan in neutered versus intact dogs.[51]

CRITIQUES OF THE DATA PRESENTED

Determining a specific cause-effect relationship is difficult, at best, given confounding factors that must be considered in any epidemiologic study. In humans, factors related to cancer development include age, gender, ethnicity, diet, occupation (often related to carcinogen exposure), environment (such as urban vs rural), and smoking, to name a few. Genetics, epigenetics, proteomics, and metabolomics are now also factored into studies of cancer etiogenesis. Rarely are these factors taken into account in veterinary studies, although research continues to expand in these areas. Selection bias is prevalent in the veterinary literature, because so many studies are conducted through teaching hospital databases. The pet population that is seen at a specialty hospital may not be representative of the general pet population: these patients are often preselected for geography, finances, and willingness to treat before referral. Pet owners who cannot afford sterilization surgery may not be able to afford treatment when a serious disease condition occurs, resulting in a perception that those animals that are intact live a shorter time. Intact animals are also likely to be referred to a specialty hospital for reproductive issues more frequently than neutered animals, resulting in a skewed population in the diagnosis database. Additionally, much of the data presented here are derived from breed-specific studies. Although these may be quite useful for recommendations for certain breeds, extrapolating to the general canine population may not be valid. These studies are also using breed clubs as their primary contacts for gleaning information. Breeders may be a different population than the general pet owner. They are more likely to be aware of diseases within certain lines and adjust their intact versus neutered animals accordingly. The response rate to questionnaires for many of these studies is also low, selecting for only those willing to respond, which may over- or underrepresent certain populations. As we learn more about the genetics and breed-specific heritability of certain cancers, we will better be able to advise our clients about the influence of many factors on the development of cancer. Finally, these studies are retrospective, which again, introduces bias and incomplete data points based on the record keeping and memories of the patients and clinicians involved. Case-control cohorts attempt to address many of the concerns mentioned earlier. Ideally, large prospective studies will be conducted (eg, the Morris Animal Foundation Lifetime Golden Retriever study; www.caninelifetimehealth.org/) that have rigorous data collection and monitoring over a long period of time to help clarify these issues.

THE PRACTITIONER'S DILEMMA

The veterinary practitioner must now weigh this information to make recommendations on the spaying and castration of dogs: both whether and when. Certainly surgical alteration can carry risks related to anesthesia and surgery, as well as sequelae such as hormone-responsive incontinence, perivulvar dermatitis, atrophic vaginitis, and endocrine alopecias.[66] Other potential problems suggested to be related to neutering, at least in the Golden Retriever, include cranial cruciate ligament rupture and hip dysplasia.[50] Several studies have linked sterilization to certain behavioral problems, as well.[51,67–69] Nonneoplastic complications with an intact reproductive system, especially in females, are also a factor. Pyometra is common in bitches over 6 years of age; vaginal prolapse may occur in young, intact, large-breed dogs during estrus; unintended pregnancy or whelping complications may ensue; pseudopregnancy and estral bleeding can often be inconvenient for owners; and finally, some behavior associated with intact females, both canine and feline, can be problematic.[66] For male dogs and cats, sexual behavior associated with roaming, fighting, urine marking, and mounting are more concerning in uncastrated animals. Benign prostatic hypertrophy occurs in more than 60% of intact dogs older than 5 years; sequelae such as prostatitis, abscessation, and urinary and defecation problems can necessitate surgical correction with associated morbidities later in life.[66]

Regarding the influence of neutering on cancer development, pros and cons for the potential increase in certain cancer types when sterilization is recommended versus the potential for overall increases in survival and decreases in certain cancer types for neutered animals should be considered. The overall incidence of the cancer type when discussing this increased risk must also be taken into account. Although lymphoma and mast cell tumor are very common, other tumor types are less; prostatic and cardiac tumors are very rare. Markedly increasing risk for a cancer type that occurs in less than 1% of dogs may remain acceptable for some clients. Breeds with high risks of certain cancers may require special consideration when discussing the risks and benefits of sterilization.

The ethics of discontinuing the recommendation for early gonadectomy, given the persistent pet overpopulation problem in the United States, is disturbing. As with other areas of medicine, the concept of personalization applies to this situation. In unowned, shelter or rescue populations, the population benefits of neutering likely outweigh any potential for increasing cancer risk. For owned animals, veterinarians will need to discuss the pros and cons for each individual and determine the best strategy for that pet based on breed, lifestyle, longevity expectations, concurrent diseases, cancer risks, other considerations for intact and sterilized dogs, and owner preferences.

REFERENCES

1. MacEwen EG, Patnaik AK, Harvey HJ, et al. Estrogen receptors in canine mammary tumors. Cancer Res 1982;42:2255–9.
2. Rutteman GR, Misdorp W, Blankenstein MA, et al. Oestrogen (ER) and progestin receptors (PR) in mammary tissue of the female dog: different receptor profile in non-malignant and malignant states. Br J Cancer 1988;58:594–9.
3. Illera JC, Perez-Alenza MD, Nieto A, et al. Steroids and receptors in canine mammary cancer. Steroids 2006;71:541–8.
4. Millanta F, Calandrella M, Bari G, et al. Comparison of steroid receptor expression in normal, dysplastic, and neoplastic canine and feline mammary tissues. Res Vet Sci 2005;79:225–32.
5. Donnay I, Rauis J, Devleeschouwer N, et al. Comparison of estrogen and progesterone receptor expression in normal and tumor mammary tissues from dogs. Am J Vet Res 1995;56:1188–94.
6. Geraldes M, Gartner F, Scmitt F. Immunohistochemical study of hormonal receptors and cell proliferation in normal canine mammary glands and spontaneous mammary tumours. Vet Rec 2000;146:403–6.

7. Theon AP, Lecouteur RA, Carr EA, et al. Influence of tumor cell proliferation and sex-hormone receptors on effectiveness of radiation therapy for dogs with incompletely resected meningiomas. J Am Vet Med Assoc 2000;216:701–7.

8. Adamo PF, Cantile C, Steinberg H. Evaluation of progesterone and estrogen receptor expression in 15 meningiomas of dogs and cats. Am J Vet Res 2003;64: 1310–8.

9. Pisani G, Millanta F, Lorenzi D, et al. Androgen receptor expression in normal, hyperplastic, and neoplastic hepatoid glands in the dog. Res Vet Sci 2006;81: 231–6.

10. Stovring M, Moe L, Glattre E. A population-based case-control study of canine mammary tumours and clinical use of medroxyprogesterone acetate. APMIS 1997;105:590–6.

11. Misdorp W, Romijn A, Hart AA. Feline mammary tumors: a case-control study of hormonal factors. Anticancer Res 1991;11:1793–7.

12. Wilson GP, Hayes HM. Castration for treatment of perianal gland neoplasms in the dog. J Am Vet Med Assoc 1979;174:1301–3.

13. Thacher C, Bradley RL. Vulvar and vaginal tumors in the dog: a retrospective study. J Am Vet Med Assoc 1983;183:690–2.

14. Herron MA. Tumors of the canine genital sstem. J Am Anim Hosp Assoc 1983; 19:981–94.

15. Aranda A, Pascual A. Nuclear hormone receptors and gene expression. Physiol Rev 2001;81:1269–304.

16. Rennie PS, Leblanc E, Murphy LC. Hormones and cancer. In: Tannock IF, Hill RP, Bristow RG, et al, editors. The basic science of oncology. 5th edition. New York: McGraw Hill Education; 2013. p. 469–500.

17. Egenvall A, Bonnett BN, Ohagen P, et al. Incidence and survival after mammary tumors in a population of over 80,000 insured female dogs in Sweden from 1995-2002. Prev Vet Med 2005;69:109–27.

18. Dobson JM, Smauel S, Milstein H, et al. Canine neoplasia in the UK: estimates of incidence rates from a population of insured dogs. J Small Anim Pract 2002;43: 240–6.

19. Bronden LB, Nielsen SS, Toft N, et al. Data from the Danish veterinary cancer registry on the occurrence and distribution of neoplasms in dogs in Denmark. Vet Rec 2010;166:586–90.

20. Merlo DF, Rossi L, Pellegrino C, et al. Cancer incidence in pet dogs: findings of the Animal Tumor Registry of Genoa, Italy. J Vet Intern Med 2008;22:976–84.

21. Benjamin SA, Lee AC, Saunders WJ. Classification and behavior of canine mammary epithelial neoplasms based on life-span observations in beagles. Vet Pathol 1999;36:423–36.

22. Taylor GN, Shabestari L, Williams J, et al. Mammary neoplasia in a closed beagle colony. Cancer Res 1976;36:2740–3.

23. Schneider R, Dorn CR, Taylor DO. Factors influencing canine mammary cancer development and postsurgical survival. J Natl Cancer Inst 1969;43:1249–61.

24. Sonnenschein EG, Glickman LT, Goldschmidt MH, et al. Body conformation, diet, and risk of breast cancer in pet dogs: a case-control study. Am J Epidemiol 1991;133:694–703.

25. Misdorp W. Canine mammary tumors: protective effect of late ovariectomy and stimulating effects of progestins. Vet Q 1988;10:26–33.

26. Dorn CR, Taylor DO, Schneider R, et al. Survey of animal neoplasms in Alameda and Contra Costa counties, California. II. Cancer morbidity in dogs and cats from Alameda county. J Natl Cancer Inst 1968;40:307–18.

27. Egenvall A, Bonnett BN, Haggstrom J, et al. Morbidity of insured Swedish cats during 1999-2006 by age, breed, sex, and diagnosis. J Feline Med Surg 2010; 12:948–59.

28. Vascellari M, Baioni E, Ru G, et al. Animal tumour registry of two provinces in northern Italy: incidence of spontaneous tumours in dogs and cats. BMC Vet Res 2009;5:39.

29. Hayden DW, Nielsen SW. Feline mammary tumours. J Small Anim Pract 1971;12: 687–98.

30. Hayes HM Jr, Milne KL, Amndell CP. Epidemiological features of feline mammary carcinoma. Vet Rec 1981;108:476–9.

31. Overley B, Shofer FS, Goldschmidt MH, et al. Association between ovarihysterectomy and feline mammary carcinoma. J Vet Intern Med 2005;19:560–3.

32. Beauvais W, Cardwell JM, Brodbelt DC. The effect of neutering on the risk of mammary tumours in dogs – a systematic review. J Small Anim Pract 2012; 53:314–22.

33. Dow SW, Olson PN, Rosychuk RA, et al. Perianal adenomas and hypertestosteronemia in a spayed bitch with pituitary-dependent hyperadrenocorticism. J Am Vet Med Assoc 1988;192:1439–41.

34. Teske E, Naan EC, van Dijk EM, et al. Canine prostate carcinoma: epidemiological evidence of an increased risk in castrated dogs. Mol Cell Endocrinol 2002; 197(1–2):251–5.

35. Bryan JN, Keeler MR, Henry CJ, et al. A population study of neutering status as a risk factor for canine prostate cancer. The Prostate 2007;67:1174–81.

36. Navarro D, Luzardo OP, Fernandez L, et al. Transition to androgen-independence in prostate cancer. J Steroid Biochem Mol Biol 2002;81: 191–201.

37. Cornell KK, Bostwick DG, Cooley DM, et al. Clinical and pathologic aspects of spontaneous canine prostate carcinoma: a retrospective analysis of 76 cases. The Prostate 2000;45:173–83.

38. Weaver AD. Fifteen cases of prostatic carcinoma in the dog. Vet Rec 1981;109: 71–5.

39. Obradovich J, Walshaw R, Goullaud E. The influence of castration on the development of prostatic carcinoma in the dog: 43 cases (1978-1985). J Vet Intern Med 1987;1(4):183–7.

40. Bell FW, Klausner JS, Hayden DW, et al. Evaluation of serum and seminal plasma markers in the diagnosis of canine prostatic disorders. J Vet Intern Med 1995;9:149–53.

41. Brodey RS, Riser WH. Canine osteosarcoma: a clinicopathologic study of 194 cases. Clin Orthop Relat Res 1969;62:54–64.

42. Brodey RS, Sauer RM, Medway W. Canine bone neoplasms. J Am Vet Med Assoc 1963;143:471–95.

43. Brodey RS, Abt DA. Results of surgical treatment in 65 dogs with osteosarcoma. J Am Vet Med Assoc 1976;168:1032–5.

44. Misdorp W, Hart AA. Some prognostic and epidemiologic factors in canine osteosarcoma. J Natl Cancer Inst 1979;62:537–45.

45. Spodnick GJ, Berg J, Rand WM, et al. Prognosis for dogs with appendicular osteosarcoma treated by amputation alone: 162 cases (1978-1988). J Am Vet Med Assoc 1992;200(7):995–9.

46. Ehrhart NP, Ryan SD, Fan TM. Tumors of the skeletal system. In: Withrow SJ, Vail DM, Page RL, editors. Withrow & MacEwen's small animal clinical oncology. 5th edition. St Louis (MO): Elsevier; 2013. p. 463.

47. Priester WA, McKay FW. The occurrence of tumors in domestic animals. Natl Canc Inst Monogr 1980;54:1–210.

48. Ru G, Terracini B, Glickman LT. Host related risk factors for canine osteosarcoma. Vet J 1998;156:31–9.

49. Cooley DM, Beranek BC, Schittler DL. Endogenous gonadal hormone exposure and bone sarcoma risk. Cancer Epidemiol Biomarkers Prev 2002;11:1434–40.

50. de la Riva GT, Hart BL, Rarver TB, et al. Neutering dogs: effects on joint disorders and cancers in golden retrievers. PLos One 2013;8(2):e55937. http://dx.doi.org/10.1371/journal.pone.0055937.

51. Zink MC, Farhoody P, Elser SE, et al. Evaluation of the risk and age of onset of cancer and behavioral disorders in gonadectomized Vizslas. J Am Vet Med Assoc 2014;244:309–19.

52. Prymak C, McKee LJ, Goldschmidt MH, et al. Epidemiologic, clinical, pathologic, and prognostic characteristics of splenic hemangiosarcoma and splenic hematoma in dogs: 217 cases (1985). J Am Vet Med Assoc 1988;193:706–12.

53. Ware WA, Hopper DL. Cardiac tumors in dogs: 1982-1995. J Vet Intern Med 1999;13:95–103.

54. Villamil JA, Henry CJ, Hahn AW, et al. Hormonal and sex impact on the epidemiology of canine lymphoma. J Cancer Epidemiol 2009;2009:591753. http://dx.doi.org/10.1155/2009/591753.

55. National Cancer Institute. Surveillance, epidemiology and end results program public use data (1973-2000). Bethesda (MD): National Cancer Institute; 2003.

56. Glickman LT, Raghavan M, Knapp DW, et al. Herbicide exposure and the risk of transitional cell carcinoma of the urinary bladder in Scottish terriers. J Am Vet Med Assoc 2004;224:1290–7.

57. Norris AM, Laing EJ, Valli VE, et al. Canine bladder and urethral tumors: a retrospective study of 115 cases (1980-1985). J Vet Intern Med 1992;6(3):145–53.

58. Mutsauers AJ, Widmer WR, Knapp DW. Canine transitional cell carcinoma. J Vet Intern Med 2003;17:136–44.

59. London CA, Thamm DH. Mast cell tumors. In: Withrow SJ, Vail DM, Page RL, editors. Withrow & MacEwen's small animal clinical oncology. 5th edition. St Louis (MO): Elsevier; 2013. p. 335.

60. White CR, Hohenhaus AE, Kelsey J, et al. Cutaneous MCTs: association with spay/neuter status, breed, body size, and phylogenetic cluster. J Am Anim Hosp Assoc 2011;47:210–6.

61. Larsen AE, Grier RL. Evaluation of canine mast cell tumors for presence of estrogen receptors. Am J Vet Res 1989;50:1779–80.

62. Bronson RT. Variation in age at death of dogs of different sexes and breeds. Am J Vet Res 1982;43:2057–9.

63. Michell AR. Longevity of British breeds of dog and its relationships with sex, size, cardiovascular variables and disease. Vet Rec 1999;145:625–9.

64. Hoffman JM, Creevy KE, Promislow DE. Reproductive capability is associated with lifespan and cause of death in companion dogs. PLos One 2013;8(4):e61082.

65. Banfield Pet Hospital State of Pet Health 2013 Report. Available at: www.stateofpethealth.com/content/pdf/Banfield-State-of-Pet-Health-Report_2013.pdf. Accessed December 17, 2013.

66. Johnston SD. Questions and answers on the effects of surgically neutering dogs and cats. J Am Vet Med Assoc 1991;198:1206–14.

67. Baumberger M, Houpt KA. Signalment factors, comorbidity, and trends in behavior diagnoses in dogs: 1644 cases (1991-2001). J Am Vet Med Assoc 2006;229(10):1591–601.

68. Kim HH, Yeon SC, Houpt KA. Effects of ovariohysterectomy on reactivity in German shepherd dogs. Vet J 2006;172:154–9.
69. O'Farrell V, Peachy E. Behavioural effects of ovariohysterectomy on bitches. J Small Anim Pract 1990;31:595–8.

The Role of Clinical Trials in Veterinary Oncology

Jenna Burton, DVM, MS[a],*, Chand Khanna, DVM, PhD[b]

KEYWORDS

- Clinical trials • Veterinary • Comparative oncology • Pathobiology

KEY POINTS

- Clinical trials in veterinary oncology serve to advance knowledge of tumor pathobiology, guide drug development and licensing, increase clinicians' ability to practice evidence-based medicine, and provide access to novel therapies.
- Well-designed clinical trials have potential to benefit both veterinary and human oncology and are essential to enhancing the practice of evidence-based medicine.
- Companion animals' owners may seek guidance from their primary care veterinarian when contemplating participation in a veterinary clinical trial; understanding the various types of clinical trials and their associated goals, risks, and benefits is important to counsel clients regarding treatment and clinical trials options for their pets.
- The goals, benefits, and risks of the clinical trial, as well as the responsibilities of the client and veterinary team during the clinical trial, should be clearly delineated through use of informed client consent documents.

INTRODUCTION

Clinical trials are used in veterinary medicine to assess the efficacy and benefit of novel chemotherapy drugs or treatment protocols, surgical interventions, and diagnostic techniques. In addition, clinical trials may be used to identify molecular targets or other tumor biomarkers and determine whether an investigational drug modifies a specific therapeutic target. Research studies involving companion animals of a particular species are most commonly designed to gain information regarding tumors in that same species and cancer therapies specific to veterinary oncology. However, spontaneously occurring tumors in companion animals are also an excellent model for many

[a] Department of Surgical and Radiologic Sciences, School of Veterinary Medicine, University of California, Davis, 2112 Tupper Hall, One Shields Avenue, Davis, CA 95616, USA; [b] Comparative Oncology Program, Tumor and Metastasis Biology Section, Pediatric Oncology Branch, Center for Cancer Research, National Cancer Institute, Building 37, Suite 2144, Bethesda, MD 20892, USA
* Corresponding author.
E-mail address: jhburton@ucdavis.edu

Vet Clin Small Anim 44 (2014) 977–987
http://dx.doi.org/10.1016/j.cvsm.2014.05.006
0195-5616/14/$ – see front matter © 2014 Elsevier Inc. All rights reserved.
vetsmall.theclinics.com

human malignancies, and clinical trials may be performed in pet animals to gain more information regarding an agent ultimately designated for use in people.[1–3] Implementation of well-designed clinical trials is essential to advance the knowledge of cancer biology and cancer therapy, in both human and veterinary medicine.

Owners pursuing cancer treatment of their pet may be presented with the opportunity to participate in a clinical trial as one of their treatment options and they may seek the guidance of their trusted primary care veterinarian when making a decision regarding clinical trial participation. Based on previous exposure to clinical trials or proximity to a veterinary center that regularly conducts clinical trials, practitioners may have variable comfort levels in counseling clients in this regard. This article provides veterinary practitioners information regarding types of clinical trials and their associated goals, describes potential patient benefits and risks associated with clinical trial participation, outlines mechanisms of patient protection and safety during a trial, and offers resources regarding available clinical trials in their area and nationwide.

PHASES OF DRUG DEVELOPMENT

Clinical trials performed in companion animals most often evaluate drugs or drug delivery, or surgical or diagnostic techniques that are ultimately designed for use in that same species. However, many cancers diagnosed in companion animals are similar in biological behavior to cancers that occur in people; companion animals therefore can serve as an excellent large animal model for evaluation of therapeutic agents before or in parallel with early testing in people.[2] Clinical trials performed in companion animals with the goal of informing human medicine are considered by physicians to be preclinical studies rather than traditional clinical trials. The term clinical trial has a broader definition in veterinary medicine and is used to describe any clinical research study that enrolls client-owned companion animals, regardless of whether the information gained from the study will be used to inform veterinary or human oncology.[4] The study end points of phase I, II, and III clinical trials, which represent the steps in the traditional drug development program, are discussed later (**Table 1**). The lack of well-defined standard-of-care treatment of many of the cancers diagnosed in veterinary

Table 1				
Phase I, II, and III clinical trials				
Trial Type	**Primary Goal**	**Secondary Goal**	**Potential Benefits**	**Potential Risks**
Phase I	Determine MTD Define DLT	Elucidate dosing schedule Gain info regarding PK/PD	Access to novel therapies Often financial incentives	Adverse events not fully known Additional blood and tumor sampling
Phase II	Determine efficacy Inform decision regarding phase III study	Better define adverse event spectrum	Access to novel therapies Often financial incentives	Efficacy not known Adverse event profile not fully described
Phase III	Compare with standard-of-care therapy	Cost and quality of life comparisons	Access to novel therapy ± Financial incentive	Unknown improvement compared with standard of care

Abbreviations: DLT, dose-limiting toxicities; MTD, maximally tolerated dose; PD, pharmacodynamics; PK, pharmacokinetics.

patients means that clients may be offered clinical trial participation as a therapeutic option for their pets earlier in the treatment process than would likely occur for human patients, who often need to fail standard-of-care therapy and standard rescue therapies before clinical trials can be made available to them. For this reason, the potential benefits and risks to companion animal participants are discussed for each clinical trial phase to allow the practitioner greater insight into the pros and cons of trials participation for their patients. The components and goals of phase 0 and IV clinical trials, which are less commonly performed in veterinary oncology, are also reviewed. A basic knowledge of clinical trial design enables a practitioner to better advise their clients as to the potential risks and benefits of study participation (see **Table 1**).

Phase I (Dose-finding) Clinical Trials

The primary goals of phase I clinical trials are to determine the maximally tolerated dose (MTD), define the dose-limiting toxicities (DLT), and delineate the safety profile of the investigational therapy. Secondary goals of these phase I trials may include evaluation of drug pharmacokinetics and/or pharmacodynamics as well as validation of potential biomarkers. The primary goals of phase I trials are generally accomplished using what is known as a 3 + 3 cohort design.[5] Patients are enrolled in cohorts of 3 and receive the drug at the same dose; if no DLT are observed, then the dose is increased and administered to a new cohort of 3 dogs. If any DLT are observed in the cohort, then the cohort is expanded to include up to 3 additional dogs. If 2 patients in a single cohort experience DLT, then the cohort is closed and the MTD of the agent is determined to be the dose used in the cohort previous to the one in which 2 patients developed DLT. Because determining efficacy against a specific tumor type is not a primary goal of phase I clinical trials, these studies are frequently open to patients with any tumor type, although there may be enrichment of specific tumor histologies if the agent is thought to have greater activity against those tumor types.

This study design is commonly used for cytotoxic drugs for which the efficacy of the agent may parallel the frequency and severity of toxicities seen with that drug. However, targeted therapies may not be directly toxic to the classic organs (bone marrow, gastrointestinal system) that have tended to limit doses of cytotoxic drugs in companion animals, and alterations in target modulation may not correlate with increased of doses of the targeted agent.[6] Therefore, it is likely more important to elucidate the biological optimal dose (BOD) of a targeted therapy rather than the MTD. The ability to identify the BOD relies on the availability and accessibility of specific biomarkers that can measure the effect of the therapy on the target. Phase I clinical trials of targeted therapies may require additional tissue sampling to determine the BOD of these agents.

Defining Adverse Events and Dose-limiting Toxicities

Determination of the DLT of an agent in phase I studies relies on careful assessment of development of adverse events (side effects) while undergoing treatment with the drug. Owners of companion animals enrolled in phase I clinical trials are frequently asked to keep close track of changes in their pets' appetites and attitudes as well as to inform the study investigator of development of vomiting, diarrhea, or other clinical signs that could be attributable to drug administration. Other critical information needed to assess the severity of the adverse event is the duration of the signs and whether medical intervention was required to treat the adverse event. Each adverse event is then graded using the Veterinary Cooperative Oncology Group (VCOG) Common Terminology Criteria for Adverse Events (CTCAE) to determine the severity of the adverse event.[7] The VCOG-CTCAE uses details about the severity, duration, and therapy required to manage the signs related to the event in order to define the grade (severity) of an adverse event. In general, grade 1 adverse events are mild and self-limiting, grade 2 are moderate and often managed on an outpatient basis with oral medications, grade 3 are severe and frequently require in-patient treatment, grade 4 events are life threatening, and grade 5 adverse events are those that result in the death of the patient. DLT are defined before study initiation and, in general, grade 3 or higher nonhematologic or grade 4 and higher asymptomatic hematologic adverse events are considered DLT, but vary for each study.

Client Considerations for a Phase I Study

Pet owners considering enrolling their pets in a phase I study should understand that the optimal dose of the agent administered is not currently known and there is a chance that the pet may receive a dose that is not effective against its tumor. In addition, the spectrum of potential adverse events that may occur secondary to drug administration often is not fully delineated for cancer-bearing animals, despite extensive safety testing in rodents and healthy, purpose-bred research dogs before study initiation. Phase I clinical trials may also require more blood and tissue sampling and can be perceived by some pet owners as more invasive than later phase studies. The potential lack of efficacy and risk of side effects are often offset by limited costs to owners once their pet is enrolled as well as financial incentives that can then be applied toward more conventional cancer therapy at the completion of the study. In addition, funds are often available to treat and manage any potential adverse events that they may occur on the study. Although this type of study may not appeal to some pet owners, it can be an excellent resource for clients who wish to pursue cancer treatment of their pets but lack the financial means to do so.

Phase II (Activity/Efficacy) Clinical Trials

Once the MTD of an agent is defined, the next step is to determine which tumors this agent may be active against and to begin to describe the efficacy of the agent; these goals are accomplished with a phase II clinical trial. In phase II clinical trials, a set number of patients are treated at the defined MTD and response to therapy is assessed at predefined intervals.[8,9] Phase II studies may be designed in several ways to assess efficacy of the agent; in veterinary medicine these tend to be single-arm studies in which all patients enrolled receive active drug (ie, no control arms and no use of placebos). Specific criteria for assessing response for lymphoma and solid tumors (**Table 2**) in dogs have recently been adopted by the VCOG and these criteria should be applied to future veterinary clinical trials.[10,11] Patients are removed from study when progression of their cancer is noted so that they may have the opportunity to pursue other therapy. Response assessment for targeted therapies poses an additional challenge as these agents may be cytostatic rather than cytotoxic resulting in stable disease (SD), which in the past has not been considered a response to therapy.[6] Evaluation of biomarkers as surrogates for anticancer efficacy may be needed to assess the response of tumors treated with targeted therapies.[6] The handling of patients with stable disease while on study should be clearly defined from the onset of the study to ensure appropriate patient care. Results of phase II clinical trials provide information as to whether it is reasonable to move forward with a lengthy and costly phase III clinical trial; if insufficient efficacy is noted in the phase II trial, investigators are unlikely to move the agent forward to compare with the current standard-of-care therapy.

Table 2 Summary of VCOG response evaluation criteria for solid tumors (v1.0)	
Characterization of Response	Definition
CR	Disappearance of all target lesion; pathologic lymph nodes <10 mm
PR	At least 30% reduction in the sum of the diameters of target lesions
PD	At least a 20% increase in the sum of diameters of target lesion using the smallest sum while on study as reference, or the appearance of any new lesion
SD	<30% reduction (PR) or 20% increase (PD) in size using smallest sum while on study as reference

Abbreviations: CR, complete response; PD, progressive disease; PR, partial response; SD, stable disease.

From Nguyen SM, Thamm DH, Vail DM, et al. Response evaluation criteria for solid tumours in dogs (v1.0): a Veterinary Cooperative Oncology Group (VCOG) consensus document. Vet Comp Oncol 2013 [Epub ahead of print].

Client Considerations for a Phase II Study

Companion animals enrolled in phase II clinical trials are all treated with the investigational agent at the MTD that was defined in the phase I study. Although many of the potential adverse effects have been identified in the phase I study, there remains a possibility that previously unreported adverse events may occur in the phase II studies. In addition, these studies are designed to determine efficacy so whether an individual animal will respond to treatment or not remains unknown. Combined with the altruism that leads many pet owners to participate with their companion animal in cancer research, benefits of participation in a phase II clinical trial may include financial incentives and/or access to a novel drug that may have efficacy against a pet's cancer.

Phase III (Comparative) Clinical Trials

Phase III clinical trials are used to compare a new drug or combination of drugs with the therapy that is considered standard of care for that tumor type. These studies are randomized, blinded, and controlled and generally require a large number of patients to be enrolled to minimize the risk of an incorrect determination that the new therapy was not different from the standard of care (type II statistical error). Phase III clinical trials are uncommon in veterinary medicine because of the cost of implementation and the number of patients needed to appropriately power these studies, but they are considered the gold standard for determining the efficacy and benefit of a new therapy compared with conventional treatment. When phase III studies are performed, they are often multi-institutional to ensure adequate recruitment of cases in a given time frame.

Client Considerations for a Phase III Study

There are few downsides to participation in a phase III clinical trial because these studies allow companion animals and their owners to have access to new therapies that are likely to have some efficacy against their tumors. Some pet owners worry about their animal being enrolled in a control arm of the study; however, patients in the control arm generally receive what is considered to be standard-of-care therapy for that tumor. If a placebo is used in the control arm, it is often combined with standard-of-care treatment or the trial may have a crossover design in which patients that initially received the placebo are subsequently treated with the active drug if progressive disease is noted while receiving the placebo.[12]

Phase 0 Clinical Trials

Phase 0 clinical trials are becoming more common with the development of targeted agents with well-defined mechanisms of action. Phase 0 trials are used to validate drug target effects and biomarkers of efficacy as well as to validate and optimize sampling methodology and handling.[13] These studies are defined by limited duration of treatment (often <7 days), a small number of patients (<15), and may require serial tissue biopsies to confirm biomarker or target modulation by the agent.[13,14] Dose escalation of the agent may occur in these studies to define the dose needed for target modulation, but these trials are not intended to replace traditional phase I dose-finding studies. Because of the short treatment duration, these clinical trials are not intended to provide a therapeutic benefit to the patients enrolled. These clinical trials may also be referred to as sampling trials in veterinary medicine because serial biopsies are often required before and after treatment to assess the effect of the drug on the tumor target.

Phase IV (After-market) Clinical Trials

Phase IV clinical trials are performed once a drug has gained US Food and Drug Administration approval; the primary goal of these studies is to gain further information regarding safety and the long-term risks and benefits of the drug in a wider population. These studies are not routinely performed in veterinary medicine.

ROLE OF CLINICAL TRIALS FOR CLIENTS AND THEIR PETS
Benefits of Clinical Trial Participation

Clients may be interested in clinical trial participation for their pets with cancer for a variety of reasons (**Table 3**). Many veterinary clinical trials provide incentives for participation; these may include treatment at no or a reduced cost to the owner or provision of a financial incentive that is provided at completion of the trial. These incentives allow clients with financial limitations to have access to therapy for their pets or the ability to afford conventional cancer treatment once trial participation has been completed. Clinical trial incentives generally are in the form of a credit at the hospital at which the clinical trial is performed, which can then be applied to additional treatment once the trial participation is complete. Participation in a clinical trial may also be of interest to clients whose pets have failed conventional or standard-of-care therapy or if the pet has a tumor type for which the response to traditional therapy is considered to be poor, such as splenic hemangiosarcoma or disseminated histiocytic sarcoma. In addition, some clients enroll their pets into clinical trials simply because they wish to advance the science of oncology with the hope of helping other pets and people with cancer in the future.

Table 3	
Benefits of and barriers to oncology clinical trials participation	
Benefits	**Barriers**

• Access to treatments not otherwise available
  ○ For pets that have failed traditional treatment
  ○ For pets with cancers that may not respond to conventional therapy
• Financial incentives
• Direct involvement in cancer research that may benefit both pets and people
	• Strict treatment schedule with possibility of additional appointments
	• May require additional blood sampling or biopsies
	• Risk of unexpected side effects, including death
	• Therapy may not be effective

Barriers to Clinical Trial Enrollment

Table 3 also summaries the potential barriers associated with clinical trial participation. Clients considering participation of their pets in a clinical trial should have full knowledge of the expectations of themselves and their pets while enrolled, as well as the risks that may be associated with participation. Clinical trial participation frequently, but not always, requires additional visits to the veterinary hospital/trials center for evaluation by the clinical trials team, and additional blood sampling and/or treatment. Pet owners should be informed of the number of expected visits, approximate length of each visit, and anticipated duration of the clinical trial. Failure to appropriately communicate the expectations of the clients during their participation in the clinical trial may result in client dissatisfaction and poor adherence to the study schedule, and consequently critical study data points may be missed. Veterinary clinical trials often operate on tight budgets and enrollment of proper patients and appropriate owners is essential to use these resources most effectively.

In addition, clinical trials may require additional blood sampling or tumor biopsies at various time points; some clients may perceive this additional sampling as too invasive for their pets. For trials investigating novel therapies, the range of possible side effects may not be entirely known. Expected side effects as well as the possibility of severe unknown side effects (including death) that could occur while on a study should be clearly outlined in the client informed consent document. This degree of unknown risk to the pet may be a barrier to participation for clients but should not be downplayed merely to increase study enrollment. Studies that are only partially funded should clearly outline client financial responsibilities before patient enrollment.

Ethics/Patient Protection

Veterinarians conducting clinical trials occasionally hear clients state that they do not want their pets to be used as so-called guinea pigs as the reason that they are not interested in clinical trial participation. Although there may be aspects of clinical research that are unappealing to some owners, it is important for pet owners understand how their pets are protected before enrollment and during the clinical trial. Means of patient protection include the following:

- Use of informed owner consent
- Appropriate trial design/good clinical practice guidelines
- Oversight by institutional animal care and use committees/clinical trials review boards
- Data safety monitoring boards

Owner Informed Consent

The informed owner (or client) consent document is a critical component to communicate goals, risks, benefits, and expectations of both the owner and supervising veterinarian while the pet is enrolled in the clinical trial. These documents should be written in a nontechnical style understandable to readers with a fifth or sixth grade reading comprehension level.[15] Informed consent documents should clearly describe the study purpose and procedures performed during the study, outline known and potential unknown risks, and as well as the expected benefit of the trial. Additional critical components of the informed consent document are listed in **Box 1**. Because signing a consent form does not necessarily imply understanding, the informed consent document should be reviewed verbally with the client and veterinarian to improve comprehension of the requirements of study participation for the client and the pet.[15] It is essential that clients have time to review the consent document and ask questions

---

Box 1
Suggested elements of consent to include in informed client consent documents

1. Purpose of research
2. Expected duration of Participation
3. Description of procedures
4. Possible discomforts and risks
5. Possible benefits
6. Alternative treatment (or alternative to participation)
7. Extent of confidentiality of records
8. Compensation or therapy for injuries
9. Contact person for the study
10. Voluntary participation and right to withdraw
11. Termination of participation by the principal investigator
12. Unforeseen risks
13. Financial obligations
14. Hospital review committee contact person

Courtesy of Morris Animal Foundation, Denver, CO; with permission.

---

regarding the study protocol before signing the consent forms. Pet owners should be encouraged to review the informed consent document with their primary care veterinarians.

Appropriate Trial Design/Good Clinical Practice Guidelines

Veterinary clinical trials need to be appropriately designed with a testable hypothesis and adequate sample size to reach the statistical power needed to ascertain differences between treatment groups. Appropriate design ensures effective use of patient and financial resources as well as integrity of the clinical data obtained. In order to provide minimum standards for the conduct of clinical trials in people, good clinical practice (GCP) guidelines were developed by the International Conference on Harmonization to protect the welfare and rights of clinical trials participants.[16] GCP guidelines define standards for trial design and conduct, data capture and analysis, as well as auditing and reporting of clinical trials with the goal of providing assurance that the study results are credible.[16] These concepts can be applied to veterinary clinical trials as well and clinical research studies should be conducted in the spirit of GCP whenever possible.

Another important component of clinical trial design is the designation of specific patient inclusion and exclusion criteria to ensure enrollment of the proper patient population as well as to confirm that patients enrolled are of good general health, other than their cancer diagnosis. Examples of common components of inclusion and exclusion criteria are as follows:

Inclusion criteria
- Specific tumor histology
- Minimum body weight
- Presence of measurable tumor
- Signed owner informed consent

Exclusion criteria
- Substage b or poor performance score
- Inadequate blood work parameters including:
  - Low platelets, hematocrit, or neutrophils
  - Renal azotemia or liver dysfunction

Adherence to this predefined inclusion and exclusion is essential to ensure the generation of the highest quality data from the clinical trial and, more importantly, ensure patient protection. For studies that require repeated blood sampling on a given day, as may be needed when evaluating the pharmacokinetics of a particular drug, investigators determine the maximal percentage of blood that can be safely drawn from a patient during a given period of time (often 5% of their blood volume) and these studies may have a minimum body weight for enrollment into a clinical trial. Studies that require tumor biopsies are likely to require that patients have a minimum number of platelets and adequate hematocrit to ensure patient safety with the procedure. Enrollment of patients that are generally feeling well is also essential for most clinical trials to ensure that patients are well enough to tolerate the sedation or anesthetic procedures that may be required for sample collection and so that any potential adverse events that may be associated with therapy are more clearly discernable from clinical signs that may be related to systemic disease or progression of the patient's cancer.

Institutional Animal Care and Use Committee/Clinical Trials Review Board

The Institutional Animal Care and Use Committee (IACUC) and Clinical Trials Review Board (CTRB) are two mechanisms for ensuring patient safety through protocol review before study initiation and monitoring patient outcome and protocol compliance during the course of a clinical trial. IACUC has traditionally overseen research animal welfare at large institutions conducting laboratory animal research and research involving companion animals at these institutions generally comes under their purview as well. Some institutions have developed specialized CTRBs to provide additional review and oversight of clinical trial protocols that enroll client-owned animals.

Data Safety Monitoring Board

Study oversight by a data safety monitoring board (DSMB) provides an additional layer of patient protection and assurance regarding appropriate study conduct and termination. The DSMB consists of an independent group of clinical experts and at least one statistician who are not directly involved with the daily study operations.[17] The role of the DSMB is to review adverse events that occur during the clinical trial and provide interim analysis of trial efficacy.[17] Although not routinely used for most veterinary clinical trials, larger clinical trials conducted in the spirit of GCP should consider use of a DSMB as another means to address patient safety.

RESOURCES

There are several resources for veterinarians and pet owners to learn more about the current clinical trials options available in their area and nationwide. It is challenging to provide a comprehensive resource list that will remain current over an extended period of time; a few of the larger, more comprehensive resources currently available are outlined here. Practitioners are encouraged to work with local specialty clinics and teaching hospitals to ensure they are informed and updated about current clinical trials in their area that may be available to their clients.

Vet Cancer Trials (http://www.vetcancertrials.org/): sponsored by the Veterinary Cancer Society. This site is searchable by tumor type and/or location of clinical trial center.

Animal Clinical Investigation, LLC (http://www.animalci.com/): an organization that facilitates veterinary specialty clinic participation in industry-sponsored clinical trials. Not limited to oncology.

Comparative Oncology Trials Consortium (COTC; https://ccrod.cancer.gov/confluence/display/CCRCOPWeb/Home): a network of 20 academic comparative oncology centers, centrally managed by the National Institutes of Health–National Cancer Institute–Center for Cancer Research's Comparative Oncology Program. COTC functions to design and execute clinical trials in dogs with cancer to assess novel therapies and answer questions about biology that are geared to inform the development path of these agents for future use in human patients with cancer.

SUMMARY

Clinical trials for companion animals are becoming more common and more accessible to pet owners as veterinary oncologists seek to expand their knowledge of tumor biology in companion animal species and improve the way they diagnose and treat cancer for these animals. Clients may seek out participation in clinical trials for their pets because these clinical studies may provide access to novel cancer therapies and/or financial incentives that can then be used toward more conventional therapy. However, many owners enroll their pets because they wish to participate in clinical cancer research with the knowledge that the information gained may ultimately benefit pets and people. Understanding of the goals, benefits, and risks of clinical trials participation provides the knowledge needed by primary care veterinarians to counsel their clients as to whether clinical trial participation is a good choice for them and their pets.

REFERENCES

1. Gordon I, Paoloni M, Mazcko C, et al. The Comparative Oncology Trials Consortium: using spontaneously occurring cancers in dogs to inform the cancer drug development pathway. PLoS Med 2009;6(10):e1000161.
2. Paoloni M, Khanna C. Translation of new cancer treatments from pet dogs to humans. Nat Rev Cancer 2008;8(2):147–56.
3. Paoloni MC, Khanna C. Comparative oncology today. Vet Clin North Am Small Anim Pract 2007;37(6):1023–32.
4. Vail DM. Cancer clinical trials: development and implementation. Vet Clin North Am Small Anim Pract 2007;37(6):1033–57, v.
5. Eisenhauer EA, O'Dwyer PJ, Christian M, et al. Phase I clinical trial design in cancer drug development. J Clin Oncol 2000;18(3):684–92.
6. Kummar S, Gutierrez M, Doroshow JH, et al. Drug development in oncology: classical cytotoxics and molecularly targeted agents. Br J Clin Pharmacol 2006;62(1): 15–26.
7. Veterinary cooperative oncology group-common terminology criteria for adverse events (VCOG-CTCAE) following chemotherapy or biological antineoplastic therapy in dogs and cats v1.1. Vet Comp Oncol 2011. [Epub ahead of print].
8. Lee JJ, Feng L. Randomized phase II designs in cancer clinical trials: current status and future directions. J Clin Oncol 2005;23(19):4450–7.
9. Simon R. Optimal two-stage designs for phase II clinical trials. Control Clin Trials 1989;10(1):1–10.

10. Nguyen SM, Thamm DH, Vail DM, et al. Response evaluation criteria for solid tu-mours in dogs (v1.0): a Veterinary Cooperative Oncology Group (VCOG) consensus document. Vet Comp Oncol 2013. [Epub ahead of print].
11. Vail DM, Michels GM, Khanna C, et al. Response evaluation criteria for peripheral nodal lymphoma in dogs (v1.0)–a Veterinary Cooperative Oncology Group (VCOG) consensus document. Vet Comp Oncol 2010;8(1):28–37.
12. Ishak KJ, Proskorovsky I, Korytowsky B, et al. Methods for adjusting for bias due to crossover in oncology trials. Pharmacoeconomics 2014;32(6):1–14.
13. Kummar S, Doroshow JH, Tomaszewski JE, et al. Phase 0 clinical trials: recom-mendations from the task force on methodology for the development of innovative cancer therapies. Eur J Cancer 2009;45(5):741–6.
14. Takimoto C. Phase 0 clinical trials in oncology: a paradigm shift for early drug development? Cancer Chemother Pharmacol 2009;63(4):703–9.
15. Jefford M, Moore R. Improvement of informed consent and the quality of consent documents. Lancet Oncol 2008;9(5):485–93.
16. Zon R, Meropol NJ, Catalano RB, et al. American Society of Clinical Oncology Statement on minimum standards and exemplary attributes of clinical trial sites. J Clin Oncol 2008;26(15):2562–7.
17. McLemore MR. The role of the data safety monitoring board: why was the Avastin phase III clinical trial stopped? Clin J Oncol Nurs 2006;10(2):153–4.

Pain Management in Veterinary Patients with Cancer

Timothy M. Fan, DVM, PhD

KEYWORDS

- Nociception • Analgesia • Cancer • Quality of life • Palliative therapy • Hyperalgesia

KEY POINTS

- Cancer-associated pain is underdiagnosed, and therefore leads to the inadequate management of painful syndromes in most companion animals.
- Early recognition of pain and preventing the establishment of chronic pain is singularly important for improving quality of life in cancer-bearing dogs and cats.
- Aggressive multimodal analgesic strategies should be instituted early in the disease course to most effectively alleviate painful sensations in patients with cancer.
- Combining pharmacologic agents, directed therapies, and supportive care strategies can effectively alleviate pain in veterinary patients.
- Effective and durable attenuation of bone cancer pain can be achieved with aggressive oral analgesics in combination with therapeutics that reduce tumor burden and suppress osteoclast activation.

INTRODUCTION

The development of cancer has become a major health concern for companion animals in the United States. In dogs, cancer is the leading cause of mortality in patients more than 2 years of age, and it is estimated that 1 in 4 dogs will die from cancer. In cats, cancer, along with renal insufficiency and infectious disease, are the major causes of severe illness and death. Although responsible for a substantial number of mortalities in companion animals, cancer exerts far greater and more pervasive morbidity in the form of cancer-associated pain, which has the capacity to diminish quality of life in most terminally ill veterinary patients.

Although the prevalence of cancer pain in dogs and cats is unknown, given the conserved biology of cancer between companion animals and people,[1–3] the incidence of cancer pain is plausibly comparable for these mammalian species. Based

Department of Veterinary Clinical Medicine, University of Illinois at Urbana-Champaign, 1008 West Hazelwood Drive, Urbana, IL 61802, USA
E-mail address: t-fan@illinois.edu

Vet Clin Small Anim 44 (2014) 989–1001
http://dx.doi.org/10.1016/j.cvsm.2014.05.005
0195-5616/14/$ – see front matter © 2014 Elsevier Inc. All rights reserved.

on epidemiologic studies in people, the incidence of cancer pain at initial diagnosis approaches 30%, and on disease progression up to 65% to 85% of human patients with cancer experience pain at some point before death.[4-8] In correlation with its high reported prevalence, pain is the most common physical complaint reported by people diagnosed with terminal cancer.[9,10] Given that dogs and cats frequently present with advanced-stage cancer at initial evaluation, it is reasonable to think that a large percentage of veterinary patients have already experienced pain during their disease progression before any medical intervention.

Cancer-associated pain negatively affects quality of life as well as many important physiologic functions, including cellular metabolism and immunity, and the alleviation of pain should be a clinical priority. In order for cancer pain to be optimally managed in pets, health care professionals and caregivers should understand the pathophysiology of pain, the different types of pain, and the recognition of pain in companion animals. A conceptual understanding of these broad areas related to pain provides health care professionals and caregivers with the knowledge necessary for the early and rational implementation of pain-alleviating strategies in veterinary patients diagnosed with cancer.

PAIN GENERATION, CATEGORIZATION, AND RECOGNITION
Pain Pathophysiology

The perception of pain is generated by the stimulation of specialized peripheral afferent neurons called nociceptors,[11-13] with the processing of pain impulses occurring in 3 discrete phases called transduction, conduction, and modulation. The initial transduction of pain begins with action potential generation through stimulation of nociceptors by noxious stimuli of mechanical, thermal, or chemical origin, and is transmitted principally by 2 types of nerve fibers: myelinated A delta fibers and unmyelinated C fibers.[11-13] Myelinated A delta fibers and unmyelinated C fibers are broadly distributed throughout the body and provide nociceptive innervations for the skin, subcutaneous tissues, periosteum, joints, muscles, and viscera. Following initial transduction, the conduction of pain follows the path of A delta and C fibers entering the dorsal horn of the spinal cord via the dorsal root ganglia, where they synapse with second-order neurons of the gray matter.[11-13] Modulation of pain then takes place in the dorsal horn, through interactions with excitatory and inhibitory interneurons. The resulting nociceptive information is carried to the brain via the spinothalamic tracts, where it is integrated, processed, and recognized as pain in multiple areas of the brain.

Although sensations of pain are normally generated following exposure to a noxious stimulus, certain alterations can result in the aberrant processing of neuronal signals, leading to an exaggerated and pathologic pain state. Examples of abnormal pain processing include hyperesthesia, which is increased sensitivity to nonnoxious stimuli; hyperalgesia, which is an exaggerated painful response to mildly noxious stimuli; and allodynia, which is an abnormal painful response to nonnoxious stimuli.[11-13] Allodynia and hyperalgesia are most commonly established in conditions of untreated or undertreated chronic pain, and result from peripheral and central alterations in the transmission, modulation, and integration of nociceptive stimuli. To effectively mitigate the establishment of allodynia and hyperalgesia, the institution of preemptive analgesia should be considered in most veterinary patients with cancer.

Pain Categorization

Although pain is a universal sensation, it can be categorized based on temporal aspects (acute, chronic, or intermittent), intensity (mild, moderate, severe, or excruciating), and anatomic origin (somatic, visceral, or neuropathic). In patients with cancer, all 3 types of pain may occur alone or in combination. Cancer pain arises from the direct invasion of tumor cells into nerves, bones, soft tissue, ligaments, and fascia. Pain can also be elicited through the distention and obstruction of internal organs secondary to tumor infiltration. Erosive and inflammatory processes elicited by cancer cells within the microenvironment can generate pain too. Cancer pain can be categorized mechanistically as nociceptive (somatic and visceral) or neuropathic in origin.

Nociceptive pain is associated with direct tissue injury from tumor infiltration and peritumoral inflammation. Perception of pain is caused by the stimulation of peripheral pain receptors residing in the cutaneous and deeper musculoskeletal structures. Somatic and visceral pain syndromes can be characterized as nociceptive. Somatic pain arises from direct injury caused by cancer cell invasion into the skeleton, soft tissues, or tendons/ligaments, often manifesting as focal and stabbing. Visceral pain arises from cancer cell infiltration, compression, or distortion of internal organs within the abdominal, thoracic, or pelvic cavities, often characterized as diffuse and squeezing. Neuropathic pain is directly related to cancer cell infiltration of peripheral nerves, nerve plexi and roots, or spinal cord, often manifesting as burning, shooting, pins/needles, or numbness. Although cancers associated with pain can be discretely categorized as either nociceptive or neuropathic, a singular tumor type can elicit pain that has blended characteristics of both nociceptive and neuropathic origin. Common tumor histologies likely associated with pain in veterinary patients are listed in **Table 1**.

Pain Recognition

An impediment for managing cancer pain effectively in companion animals is its accurate and timely recognition by health care professionals. Because pets cannot directly communicate the sensation of pain through traditional verbal cues, alternative and reliable methods to identify pain are necessary. One essential component of pain recognition is adequate communication with the pet owner.[12,14] Observant pet owners know their pets' personalities well, and can recognize subtle changes in behavior that might represent pain or discomfort.[15-18] Common behaviors noted by pet owners that might represent pain include changes in movement, posture, grooming, appetite and thirst, focal licking, drooling or dysphagia, vocalization, respiration rate, defecation, and urination patterns.

To facilitate the recognition of pain and its assessment through behavioral observations, several validated observer pain scales have been used to estimate pain in animals.[19-23] Two common standardized pain scales that are conceptually simplistic, and hence user-friendly, include the visual analog scale (VAS) and the numerical rating scale (NRS). Both are scales represented by a horizontal line, and allow for differing degrees of pain to be recorded and serially compared. There are many weaknesses with both assessment systems, but more crucial than the type of scale used is the importance of using a system that all observers understand and can use facilely and in a repeatable manner.

Despite the simplicity of the NRS and VAS assessment methods, their use by pet owners and veterinary caregivers might not be completely applicable for the assessment of tumor-bearing animals, given the distinct pathophysiology of cancer pain. To address these limitations, alternative assessment schemes have been validated for pets that include either behavioral scales or health-related quality-of-life questionnaires specific to cancer pain.[24-28] Through the use of these cancer pain–specific behavior scales or questionnaires, the objective assessment of pain and its alleviation can be more uniformly standardized in tumor-bearing pets. The recognition and assessment of cancer-associated pain collectively is best achieved through

Table 1
Common cancers expected to be painful in companion animals

Type of Cancer Pain	Anatomic Location
Nociceptive: somatic	Musculoskeletal
	Bone and joint sarcomas
	Skeletal metastases (carcinoma)
	Osseous plasmacytoma
	Craniofacial
	Oral cavity (melanoma, fibrosarcoma, SCC)
	Nasal cavity (carcinoma, fibrosarcoma, SCC)
	Skull and orbit (multilobular osteochondrosarcoma)
	Ear canal (carcinoma)
	Reproductive
	Inflammatory mammary carcinoma
	Connective tissue
	Mast cell tumor
	Apocrine gland carcinoma
	Injection site sarcoma
Nociceptive: visceral	Urogenital
	Transitional cell carcinoma
	Prostatic carcinoma
	Renal carcinoma
	Reproductive tumors
	Uterine leiomyosarcoma
	Gastrointestinal
	Pancreatic carcinoma
	Intestinal carcinoma or leiomyosarcoma
	Visceral organ
	Hepatocellular carcinoma
	Hemangiosarcoma
	Carcinomatosis
Neuropathic	Central nervous system
	Meningioma, astrocytoma
	Peripheral nervous system
	Brachial plexus tumor
	Musculoskeletal
	Vertebral body tumor with spinal cord compression

Abbreviation: SCC, squamous cell carcinoma.

combining subjective and descriptive caregiver observations along with more objective cancer pain–specific behavior scales or questionnaires.

PHARMACOLOGIC TREATMENT STRATEGIES
General Guidelines

For most pets diagnosed with cancer, pain becomes established early in the course of disease and rapidly intensifies during cancer progression. As such, pharmacologic strategies are often used in the setting of chronic pain management, in which the primary intent of intervention is to minimize the clinical consequences of peripheral and central sensitization, as well as to maintain quality of life. General guidelines for managing pain have been proposed by the World Health Organization (WHO), and can also be adapted for the management of cancer-bearing dogs and cats experiencing pain (**Fig. 1**). The WHO has specifically proposed a 3-step analgesic ladder for controlling mild, moderate, and severe pain.[29] Using the WHO ladder as a guidance tool, mild

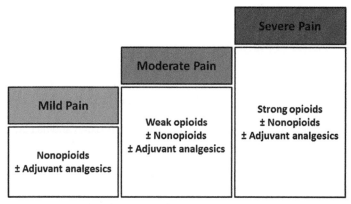

Fig. 1. The recommendations of the WHO for the stepwise pharmacologic management of pain. Given the diagnosis of advanced cancer stage in most veterinary patients with cancer, the preemptive institution of strong opioids in combination with adjuvant analgesics can be justifiably advocated for the management of pain in a substantial fraction of tumor-bearing dogs and cats.

pain is treated initially with nonopioid drugs, generally nonsteroidal antiinflammatory drugs (NSAIDs). If pain persists after treatment with a nonopioid, such as in cases of moderate pain, a weak opioid, such as codeine or tramadol, can be added. If pain is not controlled with that combination, or with severe pain, stronger opioids, preferably full mu agonists, are used. **Table 2** provides an abbreviated list of oral

Table 2 Common analgesic drugs and oral dosages for dogs and cats			
Class	Drug	Dog Dosage (mg/kg)	Cat Dosage (mg/kg)
NSAIDs	Robenacoxib	1–2 PO q 24 h	1 PO q 24 h (max 6 d)
	Deracoxib	1–2 PO q 24 h	—
	Carprofen	4.0 PO q 24 h	—
	Etodolac	5–15 PO q 24 h	—
	Meloxicam	0.1 PO q 24 h	0.1 PO day 1, 0.05 PO days 2–5, then 0.05 PO q 48 h
	Tepoxalin	10 PO q 24 h	—
	Piroxicam	0.3 PO q 24 h	0.3 PO q 48 h
	Ketoprofen	1 PO q 24 h	1 PO q 24 h (max 5 d)
	Aspirin	10 PO q 12 h	—
Opioid	Morphine		
	Liquid	0.2–0.5 PO q 6 h	0.2–0.5 PO q 6–8 h
	Slow release	0.5–3 PO q 8h	—
	Butorphanol	0.2–0.5 PO q 8 h	0.2–1 PO q 6 h
	Codeine	1–2 PO q 8–24 h	—
	Buprenorphine	—	0.02 PO sublingual q 6 h
NMDA antagonist	Amantadine	3–5 PO q 24 h	3 PO q 24 h
Combination analgesic	Tramadol	4–5 PO q 8 h	1–2 PO q 12–24 h
Anticonvulsant	Gabapentin	2–10 PO q 24 h	2–10 PO q 24 h
Tricyclic AD	Amitriptyline	1–2 PO q 12 h	1–2 PO q 24 h
	Clomipramine	1–2 PO q 12 h	0.5–1 PO q 24 h

Abbreviations: AD, antidepressants; max, maximum; NMDA, *N*-methyl-ᴅ-aspartate; PO, by mouth; q, every.

analgesics used in dogs and cats that can be easily administered by pet owners for the management of cancer pain in a home setting.

Specific Drug Classes and Mechanisms of Action

NSAIDs

NSAIDs are used to control nociceptive pain in companion animals. The mechanism of action of NSAIDs is the inhibition of cyclooxygenases (COXs). For cancer pain, COX-2 is the selective target of inhibition given its role in inflammatory pain, which is generated as a consequence of prostaglandin E_2 production. Prostaglandins play an important role in peripheral sensitization leading to a state of hyperalgesia or allodynia. Prostaglandins regulate the sensitivity of polymodal receptors, which typically cannot be easily activated by physiologic stimuli. However, following tissue injury and inflammation, the release of prostaglandins facilitate responsiveness of silent polymodal receptors.[30] Prostaglandins can also activate certain sodium channels in the dorsal horn of the spinal cord, resulting in central sensitization and the establishment of chronic cancer pain.[31] The use of NSAIDs for managing cancer pain might be particularly relevant in companion animals given the multiple tumor histologies that overexpress COX-2[32,33] and therefore have the potential for nociceptive sensitization through tumor-derived prostaglandin generation.

Opioids

Three conventional opioid receptor subtypes have been cloned and isolated: mu, kappa, and delta receptors. Opioid receptors are localized within the central nervous system, primarily in the superficial dorsal horn within laminae I to II. Within the dorsal horn, most opioid receptors are located on the presynaptic terminal of afferent fibers; however, lower densities of opioid receptors are also found on postsynaptic sites and interneurons. The mechanism of analgesia is through reduced transmitter release from nociceptive C fibers and postsynaptic inhibition of neurons conveying information from the spinal cord to higher centers of the brain. Binding of opioids to their presynaptic inhibitory receptor blocks the release of glutamate, substance P, and other transmitters, whereas binding to the postsynaptic receptor further inhibits neuronal depolarization. Opioids are readily available, can be titrated easily to desired effect, and have predictable toxicities that can be minimized preventatively.

N-methyl D-aspartate antagonists

N-methyl-D-aspartate (NMDA) receptors play a key role in central sensitization within the dorsal horn of the spinal cord following the release of transmitters from nociceptor terminals. Sustained transmitter release leads to perturbations in synaptic receptor density, threshold, kinetics, and activation, with subsequent increases in pain transmissions. During central sensitization, glutamate-activated NMDA receptors undergo posttranslational phosphorylation, which increases their synaptic distribution and responsiveness to glutamate, with resultant hyperexcitability to normally subthreshold noxious stimuli. As such, NMDA antagonists including ketamine, tiletamine, amantadine, and dextromethorphan have a role in the management of chronic cancer pain when central sensitization has been established.

Combination analgesics

Tramadol is a centrally acting analgesic and is classified as an opioidergic/monoaminergic drug based on its shared properties of both opioids and tricyclic antidepressants. Tramadol weakly binds to the mu opioid receptor, inhibits the reuptake of serotonin and norepinephrine, and promotes neuronal serotonin release. Based on these properties, tramadol is a suitable analgesic for the management of both nociceptive and neuropathic pain. Tramadol in combination with metamizole, with or without NSAIDs, recently showed clinical activity for the management of moderate to severe cancer pain in dogs and improved quality-of-life scores.[25]

Anticonvulsant drugs

Anticonvulsants are useful adjuvant analgesics in patients with neuropathic pain, as well as chronic pain with central sensitization. In companion animals, gabapentin, a structural analogue of gamma-aminobutyric acid, acts on presynaptic axonal terminal voltage-gated calcium channels to reduce neurotransmitter release. In addition, gabapentin also induces postsynaptic inhibition through evoking hyperpolarization inhibitory potentials in dorsal horn neurons through the opening of potassium or chloride channels. Gabapentin is well tolerated, highly bioavailable, and rapidly metabolized in dogs.[34] Recent studies suggest that the adjuvant use of gabapentin does not improve analgesia for the management of acute nociceptive pain in dogs[35,36]; however, other studies suggest gabapentin's activity in the management of neuropathic pain.[37]

Tricyclic antidepressants

Tricyclic antidepressants are used as first-line coanalgesic therapy for chronic cancer pain, especially of neuropathic origin. Chronic neuropathic pain can be the sequela of local nerve compression by expanding cancer cells, neuroma formation following surgical transection, radiation-induced fibrosis or neuritis, and systemic peripheral nerve damage from specific chemotherapeutic agents. The analgesia produced by tricyclic antidepressants such as amitriptyline, clomipramine, fluoxetine, and imipramine is mechanistically attributable to their actions on endogenous monoaminergic pain modulating systems. Tricyclic antidepressants inhibit the reuptake of various monoamines such as serotonin and noradrenaline, allowing these biomolecules to remain present and act centrally on descending inhibitory serotonergic and noradrenergic pathways that modulate pain transmission at the level of the spinal cord.

BONE CANCER PAIN
Unique Aspects

Bone is a living organ, rich in blood supply and nerves. Like any other organ, sensations of pain affecting the skeleton can severely decrease quality-of-life scores in companion animals. Given its principal anatomic function for bearing weight, any significant compromise in bone mineral density and quality poses a risk for severe pain and pathologic fracture.[38] Neoplasms that involve the skeleton can arise primarily from the bone, or secondarily invade or metastasize to the skeleton. In dogs, osteosarcoma (OS) is the most common tumor histology associated with focal skeletal pain[39]; however, several additional tumor types have a predilection to involve bone, including metastatic carcinoma and hematopoietic neoplasms such as multiple myeloma.[40,41] In cats, primary bone tumors are much less frequent compared with dogs; however, involvement of bone from secondary invasion is common for oral squamous cell carcinoma.[42]

The greatest density of afferent nociceptors responsible for pain impulse generation in bone is found at the periosteal surface and medullary cavity. As such, malignant perturbations affecting these bone anatomic compartments are associated with intense pain.[38,43] In dogs with OS, the generation of bone cancer pain is attributed to 2 specific host responses. First, the invasive growth of malignant osteoblasts in the bone microenvironment results in the release of chemical mediators by nonneoplastic stromal cells that in turn stimulate nociceptors and lead to the generation of painful sensations. Second, the genesis, maintenance, and exacerbation of bone cancer pain are directly attributed to dysregulated and pathologic osteoclastic bone resorption.[38,43] Based on these mechanisms of bone cancer pain generation, the most effective management of malignant osteolytic pain combines the eradication of malignant tumor cells growing within bone matrix and the inhibition of tumor-induced osteoclastic bone resorption.

Strategies to Alleviate Malignant Bone Pain

Palliative radiation therapy

Radiation therapy is considered the most effective treatment modality for the management of osteolytic bone pain in human patients with cancer, and likewise has been investigated and extensively applied for alleviating bone cancer pain in dogs diagnosed with OS.[44] The analgesic effects of ionizing radiation can be attributed mechanistically to the induction of apoptosis in both malignant osteoblasts and resorbing osteoclasts,[45] and in dogs has been documented by percent tumor necrosis assessment.[46–48] As such, ionizing radiation reduces overall tumor burden and attenuates the degree of osteoclastic resorption within the focal OS microenvironment.

Multiple palliative radiation protocols been evaluated and reported in the veterinary literature, with most dosing schemes using 2 to 4 individual treatments of 6-Gy to 10-Gy fractions. Although variable and subjectively reported in these studies, the alleviation of bone cancer pain was achieved in most dogs with OS that were treated, and ranged from 74% to 93%. Although most dogs' symptoms improved following palliative radiation therapy, the median time interval of subjective pain alleviation was not durable, and ranged from 53 to 130 days.[49–53]

Stereotactic radiosurgery

Stereotactic radiosurgery involves the precise delivery of 1 to 3 large dose(s) of radiation to a designated tumor target, which is achieved by multiple arrays of overlapping radiation beams. Similar to its utility for treating brain tumors in people, stereotactic radiosurgery has also been evaluated for alleviating bone pain associated with appendicular OS.[54,55] A nonsurgical limb salvage technique using stereotactic radiosurgery was developed at the University of Florida and initial results were reported in 11 dogs.[55] Limb use in the dogs that received stereotactic radiosurgery was excellent, and the reported overall median survival was 363 days. Advantages of this technique include limb preservation for anatomic sites not amenable to reliable surgical limb salvage, the normal tissue-sparing effects of stereotactic radiosurgery compared with conventional radiation therapy, no surgical procedures, clinically relevant pain alleviation, and good to excellent limb function.

Radiopharmaceuticals

Samarium (Sm) 153 is a radioisotope that undergoes gamma and beta decay, allowing concurrent biodistribution tracking studies, as well as therapeutic ionizing radiation delivery within a 2-mm to 3-mm deposition radius. When conjugated to ethylenediamine-tetramethylene-phosphonic acid (EDTMP), the resultant compound ^{153}Sm-EDTMP preferentially concentrates in areas of increased osteoblastic activity and binds to exposed hydroxyapatite crystals, making it a suitable radiopharmaceutical for the treatment of malignant osteolytic tumors. The use of ^{153}Sm-EDTMP has been investigated and reported for alleviating bone cancer pain in dogs with appendicular and axial OS.[56–59] Following intravenous ^{153}Sm-EDTMP administration, most (63%–83%) dogs with OS show improved lameness scores and activity levels, suggesting the achievement of pain palliation.[56–59] Despite clinical improvement in most dogs treated, the duration of pain alleviation has not been extensively documented, but seems to approximate similar durations of pain control achieved with megavoltage telotherapy. Overall, ^{153}Sm-EDTMP is well tolerated; however, side effects associated with treatment include transient decreases in platelet and white blood cell counts as a consequence of beta energy deposition within the proximity of pluripotent marrow stem cells.[58]

Aminobisphosphonates

Aminobisphosphonates (NBPs) are synthetic analogues of inorganic pyrophosphate that were initially used for diagnostic purposes in bone scanning, based on their ability to preferentially adsorb to sites of active bone mineral remodeling. At present, NBPs are considered first-line treatments for the treatment of malignant skeletal osteolysis including paraneoplastic hypercalcemia, multiple myeloma, and metastatic bone diseases in human patients with cancer.[60] The bone protective effects of NBPs are exerted through the induction of osteoclast apoptosis, which results in the net attenuation of pathologic bone resorption.[61] Although NBPs are commercially available in different formulations, the effective management of tumor-induced hypercalcemia, osteolytic bone metastases of breast cancer, and osteolytic lesions of multiple myeloma seem to require the administration of high-dose, intravenous NBPs such as pamidronate and zoledronate.

Given that intravenous NBPs are effective for the management of malignant osteolysis and associated pain in people, several prospective studies have been conducted to evaluate the potential analgesic activities of intravenous pamidronate in dogs with appendicular OS when administered as a single agent, in combination with ionizing radiation alone, or in combination with ionizing radiation and systemic chemotherapy.[62–64] The findings derived from this consortium of prospective studies collectively advocate the use of intravenous pamidronate for attenuating malignant bone resorption, augmenting weight-bearing capacity of diseased limbs, and alleviating bone cancer pain associated with focal malignant osteolysis.

Although most palliative studies have documented the effects of pamidronate, other more potent intravenous NBPs for managing malignant bone pain have also been evaluated in dogs with skeletal tumors. Zoledronate possesses 100-fold greater antiresorptive potency in comparison with pamidronate, and has the advantage of being safely administered over a shorter period of time than other NBPs. In one case report, the use of intravenous zoledronate administered every 28 days was effective for the long-term pain management of a dog diagnosed with OS affecting the distal radius.[65] In a larger study, the bone biological effects of intravenous zoledronate were evaluated in dogs diagnosed with primary and secondary skeletal tumors.[66] In this study, zoledronate was administered at a dose of 0.25 mg/kg as a 15-minute constant rate infusion every 28 days, and was well tolerated with no overt biochemical evidence of renal toxicity in patients receiving multiple monthly infusions. In 10 dogs with appendicular OS, 50% of dogs treated achieved pain alleviation.

SUPPORTIVE CARE

In addition to pain management in veterinary patients through pharmacologic manipulation and directed therapies, benefit can be derived from supportive and holistic care strategies. An emphasis on nutrition, emotional enrichment, and complementary therapies are accepted practices for the management of human patients with cancer, and similar advancements are being made for companion animals. Complementary therapies for improving quality of life in pet animals includes acupuncture, massage, stretch and manipulation, hydrotherapy, play therapy, superficial heat and cold application, percutaneous electrical stimulation, laser therapy, and pulsed magnetic field therapy. Although few studies have addressed the physiologic benefit derived from complementary therapies for improving quality-of-life scores, the excellent tolerability of these adjuvant therapies makes them an attractive addition to more conventional treatment regimens.

SUMMARY

Pain is a widespread clinical symptom in companion animals with cancer, and its aggressive management should be a priority. Education and skills can be acquired by health care professionals and caregivers to better understand, recognize, and treat cancer-associated pain. The early and rational institution of multimodality analgesic protocols that combine pharmacologic agents, directed therapies, and supportive measures can be highly effective and maximize the chances of improving quality of life in dogs and cats diagnosed with cancer.

REFERENCES

1. Breen M, Modiano JF. Evolutionarily conserved cytogenetic changes in hematological malignancies of dogs and humans–man and his best friend share more than companionship. Chromosome Res 2008;16(1):145–54.
2. Paoloni M, Davis S, Lana S, et al. Canine tumor cross-species genomics uncovers targets linked to osteosarcoma progression. BMC Genomics 2009; 10:625.
3. Paoloni M, Khanna C. Translation of new cancer treatments from pet dogs to humans. Nat Rev Cancer 2008;8(2):147–56.
4. Cleary J, Carbone PP. Pharmacologic management of cancer pain. Hosp Pract (1995) 1995;30(11):41–9.
5. Cleeland CS, Gonin R, Hatfield AK, et al. Pain and its treatment in outpatients with metastatic cancer. N Engl J Med 1994;330(9):592–6.
6. Foley KM. Improving palliative care for cancer: a national and international perspective. Gynecol Oncol 2005;99(3 Suppl 1):S213–4.
7. Jacox A, Carr DB, Payne R. New clinical-practice guidelines for the management of pain in patients with cancer. N Engl J Med 1994;330(9):651–5.
8. Sykes NP. Pain control in terminal cancer. Int Disabil Stud 1987;9(1):33–7.
9. Coyle N, Adelhardt J, Foley KM, et al. Character of terminal illness in the advanced cancer patient: pain and other symptoms during the last four weeks of life. J Pain Symptom Manage 1990;5(2):83–93.
10. Grond S, Zech D, Diefenbach C, et al. Prevalence and pattern of symptoms in patients with cancer pain: a prospective evaluation of 1635 cancer patients referred to a pain clinic. J Pain Symptom Manage 1994;9(6):372–82.
11. Lamont LA, Tranquilli WJ, Grimm KA. Physiology of pain. Vet Clin North Am Small Anim Pract 2000;30(4):703–28, v.
12. Lester P, Gaynor JS. Management of cancer pain. Vet Clin North Am Small Anim Pract 2000;30(4):951–66, ix.
13. McGrath PJ, Beyer J, Cleeland C, et al. American Academy of Pediatrics report of the Subcommittee on Assessment and Methodologic Issues in the Management of Pain in Childhood Cancer. Pediatrics 1990;86(5 Pt 2):814–7.
14. Kyles AE, Ruslander D. Chronic pain: osteoarthritis and cancer. Semin Vet Med Surg (Small Anim) 1997;12(2):122–32.
15. Bennett D, Morton C. A study of owner observed behavioural and lifestyle changes in cats with musculoskeletal disease before and after analgesic therapy. J Feline Med Surg 2009;11(12):997–1004.

16. Hielm-Bjorkman AK, Kuusela E, Liman A, et al. Evaluation of methods for assessment of pain associated with chronic osteoarthritis in dogs. J Am Vet Med Assoc 2003;222(11):1552–8.
17. Lascelles BD, Hansen BD, Roe S, et al. Evaluation of client-specific outcome measures and activity monitoring to measure pain relief in cats with osteoarthritis. J Vet Intern Med 2007;21(3):410–6.
18. Brown DC, Boston RC, Coyne JC, et al. Ability of the canine brief pain inventory to detect response to treatment in dogs with osteoarthritis. J Am Vet Med Assoc 2008;233(8):1278–83.
19. Hudson JT, Slater MR, Taylor L, et al. Assessing repeatability and validity of a visual analogue scale questionnaire for use in assessing pain and lameness in dogs. Am J Vet Res 2004;65(12):1634–43.
20. Holton LL, Scott EM, Nolan AM, et al. Comparison of three methods used for assessment of pain in dogs. J Am Vet Med Assoc 1998;212(1):61–6.
21. Morton CM, Reid J, Scott EM, et al. Application of a scaling model to establish and validate an interval level pain scale for assessment of acute pain in dogs. Am J Vet Res 2005;66(12):2154–66.
22. Firth AM, Haldane SL. Development of a scale to evaluate postoperative pain in dogs. J Am Vet Med Assoc 1999;214(5):651–9.
23. Holton LL, Scott EM, Nolan AM, et al. Relationship between physiological factors and clinical pain in dogs scored using a numerical rating scale. J Small Anim Pract 1998;39(10):469–74.
24. Carsten RE, Hellyer PW, Bachand AM, et al. Correlations between acute radiation scores and pain scores in canine radiation patients with cancer of the forelimb. Vet Anaesth Analg 2008;35(4):355–62.
25. Flor PB, Yazbek KV, Ida KK, et al. Tramadol plus metamizole combined or not with anti-inflammatory drugs is clinically effective for moderate to severe chronic pain treatment in cancer patients. Vet Anaesth Analg 2013;40(3):316–27.
26. Yazbek KV, Fantoni DT. Validity of a health-related quality-of-life scale for dogs with signs of pain secondary to cancer. J Am Vet Med Assoc 2005;226(8):1354–8.
27. Lynch S, Savary-Bataille K, Leeuw B, et al. Development of a questionnaire assessing health-related quality-of-life in dogs and cats with cancer. Vet Comp Oncol 2011;9(3):172–82.
28. Tzannes S, Hammond MF, Murphy S, et al. Owners' perception of their cats' quality of life during COP chemotherapy for lymphoma. J Feline Med Surg 2008;10(1):73–81.
29. Thapa D, Rastogi V, Ahuja V. Cancer pain management-current status. J Anaesthesiol Clin Pharmacol 2011;27(2):162–8.
30. Neugebauer V, Geisslinger G, Rumenapp P, et al. Antinociceptive effects of R(-)- and S(+)-flurbiprofen on rat spinal dorsal horn neurons rendered hyperexcitable by an acute knee joint inflammation. J Pharmacol Exp Ther 1995;275(2):618–28.
31. Gold MS, Reichling DB, Shuster MJ, et al. Hyperalgesic agents increase a tetrodotoxin-resistant Na+ current in nociceptors. Proc Natl Acad Sci U S A 1996;93(3):1108–12.
32. Dore M. Cyclooxygenase-2 expression in animal cancers. Vet Pathol 2011;48(1):254–65.
33. Spugnini EP, Porrello A, Citro G, et al. COX-2 overexpression in canine tumors: potential therapeutic targets in oncology. Histol Histopathol 2005;20(4):1309–12.
34. Radulovic LL, Turck D, von Hodenberg A, et al. Disposition of gabapentin (neurontin) in mice, rats, dogs, and monkeys. Drug Metab Dispos 1995;23(4):441–8.

35. Aghighi SA, Tipold A, Piechotta M, et al. Assessment of the effects of adjunctive gabapentin on postoperative pain after intervertebral disc surgery in dogs. Vet Anaesth Analg 2012;39(6):636–46.

36. Wagner AE, Mich PM, Uhrig SR, et al. Clinical evaluation of perioperative administration of gabapentin as an adjunct for postoperative analgesia in dogs undergoing amputation of a forelimb. J Am Vet Med Assoc 2010;236(7):751–6.

37. Cashmore RG, Harcourt-Brown TR, Freeman PM, et al. Clinical diagnosis and treatment of suspected neuropathic pain in three dogs. Aust Vet J 2009;87(1): 45–50.

38. Clohisy DR, Mantyh PW. Bone cancer pain. Cancer 2003;97(Suppl 3):866–73.

39. Chun R, de Lorimier LP. Update on the biology and management of canine osteosarcoma. Vet Clin North Am Small Anim Pract 2003;33(3):491–516, vi.

40. Cornell KK, Bostwick DG, Cooley DM, et al. Clinical and pathologic aspects of spontaneous canine prostate carcinoma: a retrospective analysis of 76 cases. Prostate 2000;45(2):173–83.

41. Trost ME, Inkelmann MA, Galiza GJ, et al. Occurrence of tumours metastatic to bones and multicentric tumours with skeletal involvement in dogs. J Comp Pathol 2014;150(1):8–17.

42. Martin CK, Tannehill-Gregg SH, Wolfe TD, et al. Bone-invasive oral squamous cell carcinoma in cats: pathology and expression of parathyroid hormone-related protein. Vet Pathol 2011;48(1):302–12.

43. Goblirsch MJ, Zwolak PP, Clohisy DR. Biology of bone cancer pain. Clin Cancer Res 2006;12(20 Pt 2):6231s–5s.

44. Coomer A, Farese J, Milner R, et al. Radiation therapy for canine appendicular osteosarcoma. Vet Comp Oncol 2009;7(1):15–27.

45. Goblirsch M, Mathews W, Lynch C, et al. Radiation treatment decreases bone cancer pain, osteolysis and tumor size. Radiat Res 2004;161(2):228–34.

46. Powers BE, Withrow SJ, Thrall DE, et al. Percent tumor necrosis as a predictor of treatment response in canine osteosarcoma. Cancer 1991;67(1):126–34.

47. Withrow SJ, Powers BE, Straw RC, et al. Tumor necrosis following radiation therapy and/or chemotherapy for canine osteosarcoma. La Chirurgia degli organi di movimento 1990;75(Suppl 1):29–31.

48. Withrow SJ, Thrall DE, Straw RC, et al. Intra-arterial cisplatin with or without radiation in limb-sparing for canine osteosarcoma. Cancer 1993;71(8): 2484–90.

49. Green EM, Adams WM, Forrest LJ. Four fraction palliative radiotherapy for osteosarcoma in 24 dogs. J Am Anim Hosp Assoc 2002;38(5):445–51.

50. Knapp-Hoch HM, Fidel JL, Sellon RK, et al. An expedited palliative radiation protocol for lytic or proliferative lesions of appendicular bone in dogs. J Am Anim Hosp Assoc 2009;45(1):24–32.

51. Mueller F, Poirier V, Melzer K, et al. Palliative radiotherapy with electrons of appendicular osteosarcoma in 54 dogs. In Vivo 2005;19(4):713–6.

52. Ramirez O 3rd, Dodge RK, Page RL, et al. Palliative radiotherapy of appendicular osteosarcoma in 95 dogs. Vet Radiol Ultrasound 1999;40(5):517–22.

53. Bateman KE, Catton PA, Pennock PW, et al. 0-7-21 radiation therapy for the palliation of advanced cancer in dogs. J Vet Intern Med 1994;8(6):394–9.

54. Covey JL, Farese JP, Bacon NJ, et al. Stereotactic radiosurgery and fracture fixation in 6 dogs with appendicular osteosarcoma. Vet Surg 2014;43(2):174–81.

55. Farese JP, Milner R, Thompson MS, et al. Stereotactic radiosurgery for treatment of osteosarcomas involving the distal portions of the limbs in dogs. J Am Vet Med Assoc 2004;225(10):1567–72, 1548.

56. Aas M, Moe L, Gamlem H, et al. Internal radionuclide therapy of primary osteo-sarcoma in dogs, using 153Sm-ethylene-diamino-tetramethylene-phosphonate (EDTMP). Clin Cancer Res 1999;5(Suppl 10):3148s–52s.

57. Barnard SM, Zuber RM, Moore AS. Samarium Sm 153 lexidronam for the palli-ative treatment of dogs with primary bone tumors: 35 cases (1999-2005). J Am Vet Med Assoc 2007;230(12):1877–81.

58. Lattimer JC, Corwin LA Jr, Stapleton J, et al. Clinical and clinicopathologic response of canine bone tumor patients to treatment with samarium-153-EDTMP. J Nucl Med 1990;31(8):1316–25.

59. Milner RJ, Dormehl I, Louw WK, et al. Targeted radiotherapy with Sm-153-EDTMP in nine cases of canine primary bone tumours. J S Afr Vet Assoc 1998;69(1):12–7.

60. Coleman R, Heidenreich A, Bell R. Managing metastatic bone disease: three case studies. Semin Oncol 2004;31(5 Suppl 10):83–6.

61. Carano A, Teitelbaum SL, Konsek JD, et al. Bisphosphonates directly inhibit the bone resorption activity of isolated avian osteoclasts in vitro. J Clin Invest 1990; 85(2):456–61.

62. Fan TM, de Lorimier LP, Charney SC, et al. Evaluation of intravenous pamidro-nate administration in 33 cancer-bearing dogs with primary or secondary bone involvement. J Vet Intern Med 2005;19(1):74–80.

63. Fan TM, de Lorimier LP, O'Dell-Anderson K, et al. Single-agent pamidronate for palliative therapy of canine appendicular osteosarcoma bone pain. J Vet Intern Med 2007;21(3):431–9.

64. Fan TM, Charney SC, de Lorimier LP, et al. Double-blind placebo-controlled trial of adjuvant pamidronate with palliative radiotherapy and intravenous doxoru-bicin for canine appendicular osteosarcoma bone pain. J Vet Intern Med 2009;23(1):152–60.

65. Spugnini EP, Vincenzi B, Caruso G, et al. Zoledronic acid for the treatment of appendicular osteosarcoma in a dog. J Small Anim Pract 2009;50(1):44–6.

66. Fan TM, de Lorimier LP, Garrett LD, et al. The bone biologic effects of zoledro-nate in healthy dogs and dogs with malignant osteolysis. J Vet Intern Med 2008; 22(2):380–7.

Index

Note: Page numbers of article titles are in **boldface** type.

A

Acupuncture
in clinical veterinary oncology, 838
Aminobisphosphonates
in bone cancer pain management, 997
Analgesia/analgesics
in veterinary cancer patients, 994–995
Anticonvulsant(s)
in veterinary cancer patients, 995
Antimicrobial agents
in veterinary cancer patients, 883–891
doxycycline, 889–890
in neutropenic patients, 883–884
afebrile, 887–888
febrile, 884–885
special considerations, 885–886
prophylactic uses, 886–887
in radiation therapy patients, 888–889
risk factors related to, 884
Antioxidant(s)
in clinical veterinary oncology, 839–840

B

Bioactive polysaccharides: fungi
in clinical veterinary oncology, 836–838
Biologic response modifiers, 927–928
Bladder tumor antigen test
veterinary version of
for canine hemangiocarcinoma, 878
Bone cancer pain
management of, 995–997
aminobisphosphonates in, 997
palliative radiation therapy in, 996
radiopharmaceuticals in, 996–997
SRT in, 996
unique aspects of, 995–996

C

Calcitrol
in clinical veterinary oncology, 839

Vet Clin Small Anim 44 (2014) 1003–1011
http://dx.doi.org/10.1016/S0195-5616(14)00117-X
0195-5616/14/$ – see front matter © 2014 Elsevier Inc. All rights reserved.

vetsmall.theclinics.com

Moving?

Make sure your subscription moves with you!

To notify us of your new address, find your **Clinics Account Number** (located on your mailing label above your name), and contact customer service at:

Email: journalscustomerservice-usa@elsevier.com

800-654-2452 (subscribers in the U.S. & Canada)
314-447-8871 (subscribers outside of the U.S. & Canada)

Fax number: 314-447-8029

Elsevier Health Sciences Division
Subscription Customer Service
3251 Riverport Lane
Maryland Heights, MO 63043

*To ensure uninterrupted delivery of your subscription, please notify us at least 4 weeks in advance of move.

Printed and bound by CPI Group (UK) Ltd, Croydon, CR0 4YY

03/10/2024

01040486-0002